Walk the Talk:
The Art of Living

DARYL VANSIER

Walk the Talk
Copyright © 2023 by Daryl Vansier

All rights reserved. No part of this publication may be reproduced, distributed, or transmitted in any form or by any means, including photocopying, recording, or other electronic or mechanical methods, without the prior written permission of the author, except in the case of brief quotations embodied in critical reviews and certain other non-commercial uses permitted by copyright law.

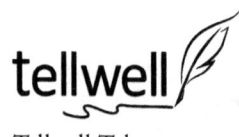

Tellwell Talent
www.tellwell.ca

ISBN
978-0-2288-9511-4 (Hardcover)
978-0-2288-9433-9 (Paperback)
978-0-2288-9434-6 (eBook)

I alone am responsible. How I live my life is up to me.

Acknowledgement

As a practitioner in the art of living the lifestyle that I have created for myself and shared in this book is the result of many influences before me for which I am profoundly grateful. I would like to acknowledge those that I know and remember: My mother for birthing me, providing for me and helping me prepare for the adventure of life. My Buddhist and Vedic teachers and their lineages of enlightened masters for educating me in how to take responsibility for my thought, speech and actions. My body-mind teachers and mentors, especially Joseph Heller, Hal and Sidra Stone, and their colleagues for teaching me how to appreciate and understand my ego-mind and facilitate this process in others. My yoga teachers and fellow yogis and meditators for sharing my path and supporting and inspiring me. My beloved spiritual and soul brothers and sisters Stefan Lacroix, Joan Matthews, Sam Giglia, Ryan Sobczak, and Erik Iversen. My ex-wife Libby Parker for partnering with me in the privilege of birthing and bringing up our beloved daughter Natalie Vansier who has surpassed our most fantastic dreams of reciprocated love and never ceases to impress us with her kind heart, mature wisdom and brilliant creativity. Her guidance supported me in creating this book and on many other occasions. I would also like to thank my dear friends Debra MacFarlane and her husband Richard Jewkes for all the beautiful photos in this book. Last but not least, I would like to thank Tereza Racekova for her impeccable work in editing this book. I thought that I had already edited enough on my own but discovered that I agreed with all of her corrections and suggestions and learned a lot in the process.

Foreword

The subtitle to Daryl Vansier's book is appropriately 'The Art of Living'. Daryl and I have been good friends for many years, and I can testify that he has indeed lived and mastered the various paths and practices described in this work.

Our friendship began back in the early 70's when he was a Zen Buddhist monk. My brother and I had developed an interest in Zen Meditation, and Daryl was our first teacher of this practice. I loved his teaching and we would go on to develop a life-long friendship. After that first lesson, I decided to become a Zen monk. During those years, and ever since, I have watched as Daryl has been inspired by, and put into practice, the various paths and ways of living described in this book. He has in turn helped countless others, some of whom have themselves gone very far in their learning and become teachers.

Like all true growth, none of this has come about easily. There have been trials, successes, as well as some very humorous episodes along the way. If I were to choose a common theme to this journey it would perhaps be

Daryl's incredible commitment and his compassion for the world and his fellow human beings. When people meet him, or attend one of his programs, they are usually struck by not only his knowledge, but also by his deep caring for their life and success.

When Daryl asked if I would contribute a forward to his book, I jokingly replied that it was not really one book, but six or seven condensed into one. This concise book presents a great overview of the wisdom gained over a lifetime of effort and achievement. Each subject can be greatly expanded. It offers a valuable introduction to avenues that bring growth and freedom. This is ever more relevant in these challenging times. I am grateful that Daryl has shared this knowledge with the world. Now it is up to readers to use whatever aspects of these teachings inspire them to enhance their own sacred Journeys of Life!

Stefan Lacroix

Spiritual teacher and guide with various career roles in the development and distribution of health and wellness products and books.

Table of Contents

Acknowledgement v
Foreword vii
Preface 1
Chapter 1   What is Life? 4
Chapter 2   What Is the Purpose of Life? 6
Chapter 3   My Moral Compass 10
    The Vision of Oneness 11
    The Power of Now 15
    The Four Agreements 20
        Be Impeccable with Your Speech 21
        Don't Take Anything Personally 22
        Don't Make Assumptions 25
        Do Your Best 28
Chapter 4   Life Force 33
    Let Food be Thy Medicine 34
    Sinful Sweets 36
    Eat Whole Foods 41

- It's Not Just What We Eat but How We Eat 42
- Circadian Rhythms 44
- Intermittent Fasting 49
- Move Your Body 53
- Yoga 55
- Benefits of Hatha Yoga 57
- Complementary Fitness Exercises 60
- HIIT 61
- Cardio 63
- Strength 66

Chapter 5 Sleep 71
- Cardiovascular Health 71
- Weight Management 71
- Immunity 72
- Athletic Performance 73
- Mental Performance 73
- Your Mood 73
- How Much Sleep Is Enough? 74
- Getting the Most Out of Your Sleep 74

Chapter 6 Self-knowledge 78
- Meditation 79
  - Reigning in the Mind 80
  - Finding Your Seat 81
  - Calming and Connecting 85
- Breathwork 88
  - Pranayama 89

- Pranayama Exercises 91
- Three-Part Breath 92
- Sequence of Eight Pranayamas 92
- Controlled Hyperventilation Technique 100

Chapter 7 Inner Work 112
- Voice Dialogue and the Theory of Subpersonalities 114
- Know Thyself 120
- Primary, Suppressed, and Repressed Selves 124
- Dreamwork 135
- Combining Voice Dialogue with Dreamwork 142
- Morning Pages 147
- The Shadow 150

Chapter 8 Outer Work 156
- Environmental Consciousness 157
- Plant Medicine 165
- Education and Right Livelihood 178
- What are My Values? 184
- Personal and Social Responsibility 186

Conclusion 191
Footnotes 193
Bibliography 197
Recommended Reading List 199
About the Author 201

Preface

I am writing and living this book for me. In this, I am no different than any other author. Whether one writes to make a living, to share one's story, to help others live a better life, or to leave something of oneself behind, it is ultimately for Oneself—oneself not as a separate entity but as part of the One Me. You, he, she, it, and they are perspectives of that One Me, the uni-verse—one infinite organism of interrelated and interdependent parts with no beginning and no end in time or space. Where do I end, and you begin? From this perspective, individuality appears to be a tenuous concept. However, most of us live our lives as though we are separate entities, ignoring our fundamental connectedness. For most of us, Oneness is a concept. Oneness does not fit into a box. It is primordial, beyond concepts. It is the substratum of all that is. No person, thing, or condition in the world of appearances can contain it or escape its imperative. Closing our eyes won't make it go away. In fact, it might draw our attention closer to its reality.

Through the guidance of my teachers and my life experience, I have learned that all suffering is rooted in the illusion of separation. Partiality and divisiveness, within and without, are the enemy of wholeness. The belief that our bodies are separate from our minds breeds disease. The belief that we are separate from our environment makes our bodies and planet sick. The belief that we are separate from each other makes us fight each other or strive to own each other. I believe that if we make Oneness our mantra, train our minds and hearts to see all that is going on with the vision of Oneness, and think, speak, and act in accordance with this vision, we can wake up from the intoxicating trance we have made our reality, witness the awesome work of art that is our life, and live in harmony with ourselves and "others."

In contrast to science, art resists definition. In the human experience, art appears to be conceived and recognized through a more intuitive process. Nature's creation is undeniably artistic and yet obedient to the scientific order. However art is expressed, it appeals to our aesthetic sensibilities and brings our attention to the extraordinary within the ordinary. Whether as a creative process or as a finished product, art inspires us to step back and appreciate. Honoring creation inspires us with a sense of purpose to our existence. Perceived with the eye of an artist, life is a work of art.

When we confer the title of "artist" upon someone, we recognize their ability to create works of art. Ability implies a skill that allows us to perform or accomplish something not just by accident but by virtue of a developed faculty honed from practice. Even a gifted artist requires the discipline of practice for that gift to manifest its full potential. Acquiring tools and instruction on how to use them from those who have experience can also be part of an artist's education, empowering one to participate in the creative process with much more ease and grace.

We are all co-creators of our life, at One with the ultimate Artist, within and without, who sees life with the vision of Oneness. This book is an offering of one who strives to cultivate this vision and apply it in his practice of the Art of Living.

1
What is Life?

Life is dynamic. Dynamism involves energy, movement, and constant change. It also involves polarity, the tension between opposing forces that holds everything together or blows them apart. We tend to attribute life exclusively to biological organisms like people, animals, plants, and microbes like bacteria and viruses, in which we can perceive movement, growth, reproduction, and decay. However, the science of chemistry and physics has taught us that nothing exists without energy; even a rock is bound together with energy. There appears to be an absence of movement. Yet, both movement and inertia are relative concepts. Everything vibrates with vital energy. The universe has no beginning or end, so it is not going anywhere in time or space, yet within its stillness, it is constantly vibrating with change. The entire universe is alive! When we say something or someone or any creature is dead, we are referring to the fact that the entity or creature no longer exists in its previously recognizable form or appearance. The creature has died, but life never dies. The river of life keeps flowing; it is never the same, but it is always there.

Life involves suffering. No surprise: life is dynamic. It is ever-changing. Polarity is at its essence, and that includes the dynamic between positive and negative. The Buddhists depict life as a wheel with various segments representing different states of existence that we pass through, and at the hub of the wheel are three creatures: a pig, a bird, and a snake, symbolizing ignorance, attachment, and aversion, respectively. The three animals are rotating the wheel by chasing each other's tails. The dynamic between them generates the chain of cause and effect, referred to as karma. It takes desire or attachment to be alive. Fear and aversion are there to protect it. What causes suffering is the illusion that we can never get to the end of it all. As the iconic Rolling Stones song proclaims: "I can't get no satisfaction." The wheel keeps turning.

2
What Is the Purpose of Life?

When I was about fifteen, I had a life-shifting experience. I was lying on my bed looking up at the ceiling of my bedroom and as often happens when one surrenders in a state of relaxation, my imagination began to wander. I contemplated the sky beyond the ceiling of our house. Intellectually, I already knew that the universe is infinite, but when I allowed myself to take it in, I couldn't, or at least my mind couldn't grasp the unfathomable. This was thinking way outside of the box, and I couldn't understand it. There was no ground to stand on, no limit to contain something for my mind to grasp. All this had the effect of triggering a feeling of being unanchored and anxious. It was the same feeling I would have when I contemplated what would happen to me when I die, so my mind took me in that direction. While I had trouble accepting the end of me when I considered the possibility of my consciousness or spirit surviving my body to exist forever, the absoluteness of forever was even more unsettling. Not only do I have no beginning, but there will be no end! Having stepped out of the box of relativity with my day-to-day preoccupations and projects that seemed to provide some sense of purpose to my existence, I could no longer ignore the big question mark at the core of my being: Why am I here? Who am I? What is the meaning or purpose of my life? On that day, the spiritual seeker in me was born. I needed to get answers to these questions. So, I spent the next thirty-five years or so looking for these answers studying philosophy and psychology, experimenting with mind-altering substances, and studying and meditating with teachers of various traditions, including eleven years of full-time practice as a Buddhist monk. The story of how that all went down may provide some interesting reading in another book, but this offering is meant to be a practical guide, so I shall fast forward to where the quest has led me.

The answer to my question: "What is the meaning or purpose of life?" was presented to me in three stages.

The first part occurred when I was interviewed for a magazine article many years ago and asked: "What is Enlightenment?" At that point in my life, I had left behind eleven years of full-time practice of meditation and related disciplines as a Buddhist monk and had been studying and practicing various branches of yoga and psychophysical therapies, which I offered in a healing center I had founded in Montreal, Canada. After years of piercing through illusions of what I or others thought enlightenment was, this word was no longer a part of my vocabulary. I could have just answered that I don't know, but I was being asked what I do know. The answer that came out of my mouth was: "When you let go of things, expectations, experiences, attachments to people, and all the projects the ego mind creates to substantiate it and ensure its survival, what's left over is enlightenment."

The second answer came from a guru with whom I spent some time in the foothills of the Himalayas a few years later. Every day he held meetings he called satsangs, during which his students were invited to express insights and questions that came up in their efforts to live consciously. At one point, Swamiji commented on how some of his students had spent twenty years studying with him and still did not find the "answer." He said that the path of self-realization does not lead you to the answer; it leads you to the question-less state. This rang true to me as our questions arise from the ego-mind. Only when we stop searching outside ourselves for the answer and tune into the fundamental ground of our being-ness—the one that simply IS—can we be free of the restless confusion of the mind.

This kind of abstract statement may trigger a skeptical voice: I might be able to tune into the peaceful ground of being when I can calm my thought waves while meditating in a safe and secure place where I am not subjected to stressful circumstances, but what if my circumstances are so challenging—whether from within or in my environment—that there is no hope of finding peace of mind in the turbulence of my suffering? In *Man's Search for Meaning,* Victor Frankl describes how he coped with almost impossible odds in a Nazi concentration camp. He was one of very few that survived three years of daily horrors, terror, and abuse in Auschwitz and Dachau. The edge of despair taught him that "Everything can be taken from a man but one thing: the last of the human freedoms—to choose one's attitude in any given set of circumstances, to choose one's own way." There was no meaning to be found for life in such abject conditions. It is up to each of us to create meaning in our lives. "Those who have a 'why' to live can bear with almost any 'how'."

Thankfully I have never had to experience the pain and anguish Victor Frankl endured, but my lifelong search for the meaning of my life has led me to a similar place. It is not a place where you can arrive. Emancipation from the cycle of suffering, the pains and pleasures of life, whether we call it enlightenment, self-realization, heaven, or the pure land, is not really a place. It is not even a state to be attained, for all states are transitory since everything constantly changes. It is an ongoing process. It is a **way.** Many prophets and teachers have offered us teachings, and there are many religions to choose from, but ultimately it is up to each of us to choose the way that works for us. The way that works contains both the why and the how. This book shares the tools that have helped make my life meaningful and worth living. Which tools you use and how you use them is your choice. We are the co-creators of the work of art that is our life.

3
My Moral Compass

The journey of life is uncharted. Google maps or GPS devices provide directions for our trips on planet Earth. Before that, we used a compass with a magnetized needle to help us navigate by orienting us around the position of True North. But what about the ultimate journey of life? If there is any journey that deserves a reliable navigation device, it is the journey of life. If we are lucky enough, our parents provide food, shelter, and basic education to keep us safe and healthy in our early years. In this, we are not much different than many other animals, but human beings also have the capacity for abstraction, allowing us to witness our conditions and reflect on them. This feeds our ego-mind and adds complexity to our basic needs for survival. Beyond our bodies, we are also mental, emotional, and spiritual beings, and our sanity requires us to integrate all these aspects. We need a moral compass to help keep us on course. Our parents, mentors, teachers, and religious leaders provide us with their input about what is right and wrong, what we should value, and the principles we can or should follow to make the best out of our life.

However, we are unique individuals, and our journey is unique. Whatever influences have conditioned our preferences, tendencies, and character, it is up to each of us to choose the fundamental principles that can serve as our moral compass as we navigate life's ups and downs and obstacles. Here, I shall share three teachings that serve as my fundamental guide.

The Vision of Oneness

The **vision of oneness** is the primary touchstone for how I wish to live my life. The universe is one. It is infinite in its multiplicity of macro and micro systems but is absolutely One. There is only one *uni*verse. The vision of oneness means recognizing that while we may appear separate from our environment and each other, that is an illusion. We are intimately connected.

I once picked up a book on a shelf in a restaurant to read while I waited for my order and opened it to a chapter titled "Personal Health" written by a medical doctor. He introduced his article by stating that the very concept of personal health is untenable. He described that while we appear to be inhabiting separate bodies, the envelope of our bodies is permeable. The holes in our nose and mouth allow the air we share and everything in it to enter the deepest recesses of our internal ecosystem. Our skin is also porous. For example, the air in our shared atmosphere enters someone's body in a remote tribe in the Amazon and eventually makes its way into another's body, drinking a latte on a café terrace in Paris. This means that our internal ecosystem and the outer ecosystem surrounding us are intimately linked, and so everyone and every creature breathes the same air. So, maintaining the health or integrity of one person cannot exclude the health or integrity of the ecosystem shared by all of us.

While this perspective is familiar to ecologists concerned about the toxicity of our earth, water, and air, our connection is not limited to our physical bodies. We are also connected energetically. Electromagnetic waves connect us through devices like cell phones and computers. Thought waves are not only transmitted through words and actions; they are also transmitted psychically. You might write off a clairvoyant's reading of your mind or your own experience of receiving a call from someone you just thought of as happenstance or coincidence, but numerous examples of human experience suggest that our psyches communicate, co-participate, and co-create within a collective psyche. The branch of psychology that focuses on such phenomena is called paranormal psychology, which suggests that it is not normal or perhaps supernatural. Science has generally focused on physical phenomena perceivable by one or more of our five senses.

However, a branch of knowledge called metaphysics includes what is called noumena: objects or events that exist independently of human sense and/or perception. This branch of knowledge has been recognized as real by mediums, psychics, and ordinary people throughout human history though not under the name metaphysics. Only recently has the realm of metaphysics been respected as scientific. When physicist and mathematician Albert Einstein developed and proved his theory of relativity, he broke through the apparent barrier separating matter and energy. His equation $E=MC^2$ says that matter and energy are interchangeable; they are different forms of the same thing. Under the right conditions, energy can become mass and vice versa. This important development led to quantum mechanics, which describes the world at the microcosmic level of subatomic particles and waves. One of the mysteries that it has uncovered is "the observer effect," which posits that "the outcome of a quantum experiment can change depending on whether we choose to measure some property of the particles involved." This was deeply troubling as it seemed to undermine the basic assumption behind all science: that there is an objective world out there, irrespective of us. If the way the world behaves depends on how—or if—we look at it, what can reality really mean?[1] So, to put things more simply, our world—the universe—has both a relative and absolute reality. At the relative level, we and objects appear to be separate. At the absolute level, we are one interdependent Me.

At the relative ego level, we are separate individuals, each with our own story and the personalities we have developed to cope with life's challenges. As soon as we became conscious of being separate entities with needs and fears, ego was born. As we discovered ways of avoiding pain and meeting our needs at the most

---

[1] http://www.bbc.com/earth/story/20170215-the-strange-link-between-the-human-mind-and-quantum-physics

basic levels as infants, this developed into habitual behaviors that appeared to help or promised to help. These habits and characteristics became personalities that view the world and others from their particular and unique perspective. We need our egos for our bodies to survive; this consciousness of our separateness enables us to get what we want and avoid what we don't want. The problem is that the ego becomes more concerned about protecting itself than just ensuring the survival of the human organism. That's when suffering happens.

The root of all suffering is the sense of separation. Perceiving ourselves as separate from nature brings fear of nature and its creatures. It also breeds abuse of nature and the consequences of that abuse. Perceiving ourselves separate from our human brothers and sisters breeds attachment, rejection, longing, envy, jealousy, anger, hate, lust, mistrust, judgment, paranoia, lying, competitiveness, greed, and all their consequences. This sense of separation often extends to collective separation when we join with others to separate from another group, nation, political party, race, or affiliation that we perceive as too different, not sharing our values and agendas, or threatening what we are attached to or identify with. This leads to disharmony, conflict, dysfunctionality, and wars.

Inner conflict, anxiety, depression, loneliness, low self-esteem, insecurity, frustration, and despair stem from a sense of separation within—a lack of connection with our essential Me that is not identified with the conflicting agendas of the different parts or selves within. This will be described more thoroughly in the chapter on subpersonalities and Voice Dialogue. What can be stated here is that reminding ourselves that we are one with everyone and everything encourages inner and outer harmony and fosters love, compassion, kindness, empathy, peace, trust, honesty, and clear communication. The two other teachings that make up my moral compass emanate naturally from this vision of Oneness and help me cultivate it.

The Power of Now

Our sense of separation or apart-ness involves experiencing our infinite universe in terms of its finite parts. This division occurs in both time and space. Physical reality, whether perceived as a state or as movement from one place to another or one object relative to another, requires the interdependent dimensions of time and space. Time is just as much a dimension we move through as spatial dimensions are dimensions, we move through. So, the cultivation of Oneness necessarily includes our relationship with time.

You have most probably experienced how time can seem to stand still, or it can fly. We also know that if we are moving alongside another object at the same speed, it seems that we are not moving. Objective reality is only as real as the variables that affect our perception of it.

So, when we speak of how the suffering of life is rooted in the sense of separation, we must include how we are affected by the passage of time. How does our perception of time make us feel separate or less connected? Firstly, the three ways we separate time—past, present, and future—are an illusion created by our minds. With Einstein's theory of relativity and subsequent discoveries, it has been established by the laws of physics that time and space are interdependent dimensions. How events play out depends on the reference point of each individual. Without going into complicated scientific experiments and theories of which I know little, I would like to share with you what the experiment of life has taught me about my relationship with the past, present, and future. Whatever I have understood intellectually about how our separating time into past, present, and future is an illusion, it has not changed the reality that I do not suffer when I am living in the present moment.

Before I go on, I need to qualify my use of the word suffering. The Buddhist teachings distinguish physical pain and mental/emotional suffering. In other words, we can experience physical pain without suffering from it. This is not to say that physical pain does not contribute to mental suffering. Mental suffering can also increase physical pain. The following example will help to illustrate this. In one of my meditation classes, I had a student who had informed me that she could not sit in one of the classic sitting postures on the floor because she had been operated on for a serious back problem, and several of her vertebrae were held together with steel rods called Harrington rods. I told her she could meditate sitting in a chair, but I was somewhat concerned about how it would go with her.

During the sharing at the end of the class, some of the students who were new to the experience of meditation described how they had struggled with discomfort and, in some cases, had to move and break posture during the relatively short sitting period of about twenty minutes. When it came time for the student sitting in the chair to share her experience, it was clear that she had not suffered at all, and this was entirely believable as she had not moved during the sitting. She said that she had never been without physical pain since the surgery, but this did not in any way interfere with her meditation. In fact, we learned that she had been meditating for years. It was evident to everyone in the room that she was probably the most peaceful and joyful person in the room. This was an inspiring example of how the meditating mind can alter the experience of physical pain such that one need not suffer from it. It was also clear that it is not the degree of physical pain that determines the degree of mental suffering, as others present suffered with little or no physical pain. We will look more closely at what happens with our mind when we meditate in the chapter on meditation, but what I can say here is that it has to do with how we experience the passage of time. Simply put, meditation is practicing presence of mind.

The mind tends to wander. It will either remember things from the past or anticipate events in the future. Even in the rare moments when we are focused on our present experience, the mind will associate something in the experience with something that has happened before and reflect on that, or it will make plans for the future based on the present experience. To fully enjoy anything, we need to be fully present with it. As soon as we separate from our experience by wanting to keep it or by comparing it to another experience, we are no longer present or at one with it. At that moment, we lost our enjoyment of the present moment and opened the door to suffering. This is why the Buddhists view both pleasure and pain as suffering. Running after pleasure and away from pain is part of the cycle of suffering.

It is not what we desire or fear that causes our suffering. It is our mind going forward or backward in time. In fact, our mind does not have to go far for us to suffer. Of course, it is useful for us to recall the past, to learn from our experience and thus improve our capacity to make the best of the present. However, our past experiences have etched grooves into our memory and each cell of our body so we can literally carry the pain of the past, which will also interfere with our capacity to enjoy the present moment. Like water flowing through pre-formed channels, our minds flow into familiar grooves or ruts, and habits are formed, then sets of habits become characters or personas that predetermine our experience depending on which one is triggered by a particular experience or situation. In his preeminent book *The Power of Now*[2], Eckhart Tolle calls this the pain-body.

---

[2] *The Power of Now,* Eckhart Tolle. Namaste Publishing 1997 Vancouver, B.C., Canada and New World Library 2004, Novato, California, USA. This is one of the essential books I have included in my recommended reading list to accompany this book both for its accessible instruction and the inspiration you will receive to practice living in the moment.

Projecting our reality into the future is also useful to help us plan appropriate and efficient courses of action and prevent mishaps, but it can also compromise our capacity to enjoy the present moment. To understand this process, let us look at our experience of desire and fear. Desire and fear are, in essence, natural and useful functions, but our mind can modify their expression in ways that cause suffering. Anxiety, phobias, and paranoia are modifications of fear and desire in human experience. Fear, in its purest expression, is our nervous system alerting us to the presence of danger. Desire wants to keep us alive. Anxiety is a little more complicated. Though often confused with fear, it is often rooted in desire. We get anxious about not being able to get what we want or need or losing something we have. Our "fear" of a negative outcome in the future is more accurately an anxiety based on being attached to a desired positive outcome or expectation. Some examples of this and how to manage this tendency will be described in the next chapter. Phobias are similar to anxiety but more akin to fears because they involve a perceived threat, for example, a fear of snakes, crowds, closed spaces, or huge open spaces. Paranoias are more opinion-based—distorted illusions created by the mind. What these have in common is how our imagination can create modifications of our natural functions of fearing, desiring, and reasoning that cause suffering.

Living in the present moment is more challenging than it may sound, as we can only be as present as our consciousness allows us to be. The mind busies itself with recalling or imagining the past and projecting it into the future. It also accumulates impressions of our experience. The energies that are accumulated in our storehouse of memory are not all available to our capacity to recall, but they are still alive. The impressions of our past experiences are present in every cell of our body-mind. Whatever is hidden in the shadows of our body-mind is outside of our conscious control and, therefore, profoundly influences our capacity to be truly present. In the chapter titled Inner Work, we shall examine the theory of subpersonalities and learn how we can dig below the surface to recruit and integrate all the members of our inner family into the work of becoming fully conscious.

The Four Agreements

Having been brought up in a Judeo-Christian environment, the Ten Commandments served as my first moral code in this life. Since then, I have investigated others from other traditions. The moral code that I have found most user-friendly and yet profound in its implications in support of the vision of Oneness comes from the Toltec teachings[3]. It is called The Four Agreements, or at least that is the title made popular today by Don Miguel Ruiz, a medical doctor who was trained in the teachings of the ancient Toltec tradition by his Mexican mother Sarita after a severe car accident turned his life around. He wrote a tiny book containing what I consider a comprehensive

---

[3] https://www.susangregg.com/toltec-tradition/

guide to creating a fulfilling life: *The Four Agreements*.[4] The word *agreements* is appropriate. They are not commandments imposed from above to be obeyed lest ye be punished but rather guidelines that help us take responsibility for making the best of our lives. I highly recommend that you read this precious book and I have included it in my *Walk the Talk* reading list, but I shall share a brief outline here.

Be Impeccable with Your Speech

This is the first Agreement. The key word here is *impeccable.* The word means flawless but originates from the Latin word *peccare*, which means liable to sin. The English Biblical word *sin* has come to be associated with guilt for transgressing divine commandments. However, the Latin version of the Bible used the word *peccatum*, meaning error or missing, and the Greek version used the word *hamartia*, denoting the act or state of missing the mark. It is an archery term. It takes true aim for the arrow to hit the mark. To depart from truth is to lie to one side or the other, to err from the straight and narrow. Being impeccable with your speech is not just about not telling an outright lie. It is about not lying to one side or the other or deviating from the proper use of speech. Anything we say that creates a sense of separation or partiality is a misuse of speech.

---

[4] *The Four Agreements: A Practical Guide to Personal Freedom*, Don Miguel Angel Ruiz, 1997 Amber-Allen Publishing; San Rafael, California

When we judge others, when we slant our words to manipulate others for our own agendas, when we boast to make ourselves look good, when we hurt others with our words, when we gossip, whether with conscious intent to denigrate others or to secure membership in a group, or even idly repeat things we have heard to incite interest or fill the space with words, we are departing from impeccable speech. Untrue speech lacks integrity. Integrity is about wholeness. Whatever divides, hurts, intoxicates, attempts to seduce, misrepresents, or tricks to win something for oneself lacks integrity. Practicing impeccable speech is not just for others but also oneself. Lying to ourselves, making ourselves feel small, is also a misuse of the precious gift of speech. Practicing impeccable speech must start with the unspoken word. We need to be aware of our mind chatter because every word uttered originates in our mind. What is my intent for wanting to say something? When a voice inside me expresses something partial, it needs to be balanced with the perspectives of other parts of me so that it does not compromise my well-being or connection with others. Often what we project onto others stems from unexamined or unintegrated voices within. Impeccable speech does not harm self or other. The commandment, *thou shalt not kill,* is implied in the first agreement because right speech supports life and love.

Don't Take Anything Personally

This is the second Agreement. Usually, we understand this to mean not allowing a slight or criticism from another hurt our feelings. Indeed, that is a part of it, but it is just as much about not becoming identified with a compliment or praise from another. When we identify with a negative or positive comment or action directed towards us from another, it feeds an illusory and, therefore, fragile identity or aspect of our ego. The problem lies in that part of us clinging to what is someone else's projection. When we take something personally, we have done just that; we have taken it to be our own. If I greet the cashier at the grocery store and they don't respond, it does not mean I have done something wrong, nor that they have a problem with me or are mean or hostile. Perhaps they are preoccupied with something that happened to them that day, or they woke up on the wrong side of the bed, or they have a different way of interacting with others than I do. Whatever it is, I do not have to make it my problem. However, let's be clear: If I perceive it as their problem and I get an energetic charge judging them for their problem, I have made it my problem. I have taken it personally.

Similarly, if someone expresses admiration for something I have accomplished or a quality they perceive in me, and I buy into it or take delight in it as in getting a false sense of security or self-worth from it, or worse, I use it to influence that person or others to push an agenda, ambition, or fantasy I might have, then I have taken it personally. A part of me, some persona in me, has appropriated that event for its purposes. This does not mean that I should not accept or appreciate a compliment from another person. It just means not clinging to it. It is their perception. This agreement dovetails with the first agreement.

For example, if I tend to ally myself with those who agree with me, speak my language, and share my political beliefs and exclude those who do not agree with me, speak my language, or share my beliefs, then I am taking things personally because I am writing off a person just because they do not agree with me. Whereas, if I learn to listen with a critical but open mind to another point of view, without taking it personally, I may adjust my perception and perhaps learn to speak their language, and then we may find common ground and expand our perspective. It should be mentioned here, too, that not taking things personally does not mean that we should become numb and feel no emotion. If someone criticizes me for something that I have said or done or did not say or do when I should have, some vulnerable part of me may be triggered, so it has touched me personally, but I don't have to cling to it by feeling defeated or defending myself or fighting back with a countercriticism. It is an opportunity to improve any behavior that limits my capacity to participate more harmoniously in my relationships with others. I can also witness a part of myself appreciating a compliment or praise and feeling good about it while remaining conscious that while that part of me can gain more confidence, it is not essential for my general self-worth. Not taking things personally helps us become more aware—to stand apart—not only from the expressions of other persons but also from the persona within us that has its way of experiencing reality. Ironically, standing apart or separating from personal identification results in more capacity to embrace all the parts of the big Me. The chapter on Voice Dialogue and subpersonalities will explore this perspective more in-depth.

Don't Make Assumptions

This is the third Agreement. We are all conditioned beings. We don't get an instruction manual before we emerge from our mother's womb as a separate vulnerable human being and experience the staggering change of taking our first breath, and there are many experiences to follow. Learning from our experiences is an inescapable imperative if we are to survive physically, mentally, emotionally, and spiritually. If we are lucky, we learn many valuable lessons from our parents, teachers, guides, and mentors. Much of our learning is also a matter of trial and error. Whether we try something we have been shown or initiate our own experiment, the outcome will influence our attitude toward our experience. If the outcome is positive, we are likely to repeat it, make a habit of it, and believe in it. Curiously, we can make a habit of it even when we are not successful in achieving the desired result. Why would we do that? Everything we have learned or experienced leaves an impression on us and conditions how we react or respond to a new experience. If we have received a favorable impression about someone by following their advice and having positive results in the past, we may be motivated to keep trying something they suggest that has never worked for us, believing that eventually, it will.

We can even make a habit of acting in ways that consistently yield negative results without someone else influencing us. Perhaps when we were still babies, we got our mama's attention by making a lot of noise, and she came to comfort us or feed us. However, after a while, she or both parents reacted with anger or scolding because it became excessive. The negative attention-getting behavior may eventually be modified, but the earlier habit is already imprinted and may continue to condition our strategies to get attention even when that has negative results. It also has the compound effect of prejudicing the response of those close to us whose attention we might most want to get.

Our pre-conditioning contributes to our making assumptions. When something resembles something we have experienced before, the mind can quickly jump to conclusions. For example, you are going out to try a new restaurant, and all the restaurants you have gone to in your area allow you to pay with a credit card, so you want to travel light and not bring cash. A little voice whispers that maybe you should call ahead to ask if they accept credit cards, but it's reasonable to assume that you don't need to bother, so you don't. Sure enough, when it's time to pay, you discover that they don't take credit cards. Now that isn't a dire consequence, but let's say you are visiting another city and you are from a place that allows people, either officially or not, to jaywalk. You see an opportunity to take a shortcut and assume the oncoming car will slow down. It doesn't, and you end up on a stretcher in an ambulance or worse. I am sure you can imagine many situations where you have made assumptions based on past experiences in similar circumstances.

Like the other Agreements, making assumptions impacts your efforts to practice the other Agreements. If you make assumptions about what someone is saying or is about to say based on your past experiences with that person or others, you will likely err from being impeccable with your speech. Similarly, making an assumption about the implications or intent of another's words or actions towards you increases the chance that you will take it personally. What is interesting about the Four Agreements is that this also works the other way around. Impeccable communication is about listening and keeping an open mind. So, if you are conscious and responsible in your conversations with others, you are less likely to make assumptions or take things personally.

Making assumptions is a precursor to having expectations. I was trying to think of an example of this when I received a text message from a friend who had invited me for dinner but had to postpone. She did not have time to prepare due to having spent most of her day following a lead to find her beloved dog that had gone missing a few months earlier. This was not the first time she had followed up on leads as her community is small, and she had reached out in every way possible through neighbors, social media, and friends many times, and each time she was sure that she had finally struck gold. Her continued efforts were commendable, and I had several times encouraged her to keep the faith. The problem was that it was easy for her to make reasonable assumptions based on the information she was getting, which contributed to her high expectations.

What was compounding her suffering and possibly interfering with the manifestation of what she desired was that each time, her expectations were so high, and then they were disappointed. So, I wrote her back: "If I may be so bold to make a suggestion: Keep the faith but with no expectation." She immediately responded: "You may be so bold. My expectations ratcheted up 1000%. I 'knew' she would be in my arms tonight. Thanks for the note!" This is also a good example of how our desires fuel our assumptions. I want to be very clear here. I am not against desiring. Without desire, there is no life. One of my teachers proclaimed: "The problem is that people don't desire enough, and they settle for gratifications or partial desires. It takes big "D" Desire to reach fulfillment." Faith and desire are very connected. Desires for things or experiences feed expectations and consequent disappointments. Faith is also a manifestation of desire to support life, but it is always hopeful—not expecting nor disappointed. Not making assumptions helps nourish the faith-mind. Life is much more enjoyable when you have no expectations.

Do Your Best

The fourth Agreement also supports practicing the other three Agreements, and **do your best** is another way to say **keep the faith**. For many, faith has come to mean believing that a superior entity will take care of things. You have probably heard the saying "God helps those who help themselves." Perhaps Gautama Buddha was responding to followers deifying him when he instructed them not to believe anything he said without testing it in practice. At the moment of his great awakening or enlightenment, the Buddha supposedly uttered: "I alone am responsible." "I alone" means I all-One, no other, no one else. No one else but me is responsible. This is good news. Some people don't like the concept of karma because they believe it means they are to blame for what befalls them. Simply put, karma is cause and effect. As ye sow, so shall ye reap.

Feeling sorry for ourselves or blaming ourselves or another for our misfortune is forgetting that if I alone am responsible, I have the power to make my life better. If I do my part as best I can, I trust that things will work out sooner or later. That is my understanding of faith. Faith and grace are a dynamic duo. The Japanese Buddhists call it *joriki* and *tariki*. Faith or *joriki* is what I do, my efforts. Grace or *tariki* is what I receive, and that inspires my efforts. If God is the One and Only, that means God is none other than you or me. Whatever is happening is part of my reality. Ultimately, I am responsible. It is up to me to respond as best I can to what is. Doing my best is not a partial effort. That would not be believing in, trusting, and honoring my full potential.

Ironically, doing my best is not trying or expecting to do more than my best. If my inner critic chastises me for falling short in my efforts, and I submit to that voice and either try too hard or give up trying altogether, that is not doing my best. I once resolved not to judge anyone, including myself, for seven days. Try it sometime. It's not as easy as it may sound. I was not successful, but I learned a lot about what it means to do my best. The more I tried to perfect my practice of not judging, the more I was tested. When an apparently judgmental thought would arise, I would not only have to discern whether I was judging another person but also whether I was being too critical of my own performance of the practice of not judging. Letting go of that judgment meant that I had to go easier on myself.

Your best and my best are not the same. Doing our best is unique to each of us. This is one of the great challenges in designing a progressive and effective education system. While there are common values and interests that we can agree on, we also have very individual interests, inclinations, and even values as students, and our teachers may not share our perspectives. What kind of grading system can fairly evaluate each student's knowledge of the subject being graded? We may differ in our perspectives and express these perspectives differently from our fellow students and teachers, so the "right" answer, according to the teacher or textbook, may not accommodate a valid perspective that differs. I once heard the dean of my Alma Mater university proclaim that the primary goal of educators is to teach critical thinking. Imposing commonly held beliefs and categorizing people's progress by how they compare with the rest of the group in their test responses can be limiting and compromise the goal of developing critical thinking. I once did an extensive bodywork training called Hellerwork that involved a combination of deep tissue manipulation, movement re-education, and dialogue. What attracted me to Joseph Heller's approach as compared with another similar training I was considering was his response to my telling him that I was concerned about having to do six months of "auditing" in another training, which involved passively observing others being trained as a prerequisite to the phase of actual hands-on practice. He did not believe in this approach and shared his vision of what education should be.

The word education comes from the Latin *exducere*, which translates literally as "to lead out of." Education should not just try to put ideas and information into students' heads. It should be more about drawing out knowledge from each student, helping them discover and create with what they discover. Joseph Heller informed me that he did not believe in examinations, so there were no tests to pass in his training. Though this seemed encouraging to me initially, it became a challenge later in the training. There were a few people in my training group who I believed were not qualified to properly represent the work practicing with real clients, and I thought that if they were to be evaluated by an examination, they would surely not pass. As it turned out, they "weeded" themselves out of the work. One quit before the end of the training and the other abandoned his professional practice not long after starting.

Another important lesson I learned in this training was how effective it was to allow each student to learn and express their learning in their own way. This means that our best cannot be measured up against another's accomplishments. This does not mean that we cannot benefit from the example of others. Others can provide us with tools and skills that will help us expand our potential to manifest what we value. Perhaps even more important than specific tools and skills, the example of others can demonstrate the possibility that we can do it too. We are not required to become who they have become, but their example can inspire and encourage us to venture beyond the "box" of beliefs, habits, and attitudes that limit our capacity to manifest our unique potential.

A final thought: Doing our best is not just about working hard. In fact, this attitude can work against us. The pusher inside us wants us to push beyond our weaknesses, and our inner critic calls us lazy. However, there is tremendous power locked up in our so-called weaknesses if we allow ourselves to get to know them and make friends with them. Pretending that they are not there is closing the door. Energy cannot be diminished, but it can be blocked. When energy is blocked, it looks like weakness. We need to be gentle enough with ourselves to embrace our vulnerabilities and include them in our quest to express our full potential. Laziness is a superficial label that we put on a lack of motivation. When we lack motivation, it is either that what we are trying to do is not appropriate to where we are in our process or that it is not aligned with who we are. We shall explore this in more detail in the chapter on inner work.

4
Life Force

Perhaps the most fundamental requisite for a fulfilling life is a healthy body and mind. What does it mean to be healthy? Health is a word that stands in fragile opposition to its opposite: sickness. It usually refers to a body that is free of disease and functions well. However, a body that functions well is sensitive to toxic conditions and reacts appropriately to alert us, fight off destructive intruders, or restore homeostasis if its integrity has been compromised. So, when we are feeling sick, we are actually experiencing symptoms of the body's efforts to heal itself. Like happiness, health is a relatively ephemeral experience, more of a dynamic process than a fixed state. Our body maintains itself brilliantly without our conscious participation but only for so long if we don't listen to its signals and do our part to give it what it needs to continue to perform its functions effectively.

The most essential need of any living organism is life force or what the yogis call *prana,* and what ancient Chinese medicine and the Taoists call *chi. Prana* has sometimes been translated as breath. Though breath is our primary source of prana, prana refers to life force or life energy, and it is found not only in the air around us but also in our food, in the earth beneath us, in the water we drink and bathe in, and in the rays of the sun. Energy is abundant, but it is more or less available to us, depending on our capacity to process it. Our body-minds are amazingly sophisticated energy processors, and like any machine, one needs to know how to use it to get the most out of it. We come equipped with an innate program, like software in a computer, that allows our organism to carry on basic but incredibly complex functions and includes basic instincts to help us interact with our environment and others and to build on that experience to develop a sophisticated matrix of intelligence. However, we need to educate ourselves to avoid toxic substances in our environment, avoid toxic behaviors and habits that compromise the integrity of this incredible energy processor that we so often take for granted, and properly fuel this complex organism so that it will function at its highest capacity and without burning itself out.

Let Food be Thy Medicine

Hippocrates, the great physician considered the father of medicine, said, "let food be thy medicine." Unfortunately, modern medical practice seems to have forgotten this wisdom. Doctors are primarily trained to focus on repairing our bodies with surgery or treating diseases with synthetic drugs. Granted, technology has evolved to equip practitioners with sophisticated diagnostic and surgical machines, and this certainly comes in handy when we have been injured or are suffering from various diseases. The problem is that none of this encourages the patients to educate themselves and take responsibility for their own health beyond showing up for annual check-ups or rushing to the doctor or hospital when they have a problem. There will probably always be a need for doctors or other medical professionals to help us take care of ourselves, but it is evident that despite the billions of dollars spent on the medical system, there are still many casualties and plenty of people suffering from chronic illness. This would not be the case if we, the patients, knew how to care for our body-minds. Many people take better care of their cars than their own bodies. They wouldn't pour Coca-Cola into their gas tank but have no problem putting it into their bodies. Our first responsibility is to feed ourselves properly, which doesn't just mean avoiding the more popular junk foods.

Few doctors are trained in what I consider essential medical knowledge: the art of nutrition. Doctors do not totally deny this aspect of health, but it is usually delegated to nutritionists in the medical system that few people consult unless assigned to them when they end up in a hospital. I won't comment here on these nutritionists' competency except that recent scientific research has shown that much of what the nutritionists within the medical system have been taught is outdated and not in agreement with current findings. Of course, with all the different diets we have been exposed to, we know that nutrition is a controversial subject, but part of educating ourselves is to think critically and investigate by personal experience. This is one important area to avoid making assumptions about.

I am not a nutritionist or biologist, but I have been interested in nutrition for about fifty years. I have informed myself through books and the internet and used my own body as a laboratory for experimenting with numerous dietary regimens, including vegetarian, vegan, raw food, macrobiotic, primal or paleo, and many variations of these, including specific nutritional protocols to help my body heal particular issues rather than control symptoms with synthetic drugs. It is still an ongoing experiment for me; therefore, I won't recommend any particular dietary program, but I will share what I have found these various approaches agree on and to which my body has responded well.

Sinful Sweets

The expression "sinful sweets" is an ironic way to make sugar seem harmless and acceptable, and this is understandable as it is ubiquitous in our food supply, and our consumption of it is excessive. A quick search online will show several different results in terms of how much the average first-world person consumes a day and differing opinions of the recommended daily limit, but all sources resoundingly agree that the average consumption is over the limit of what is considered healthy. Many findings are based on added sugar and do not consider the amount of sugar that naturally occurs in our foods. Most food has some sugar or carbohydrates in it. We all need some carbohydrates to sustain our bodies, but the diet of most first-world countries is excessive in the sugar department. The main reason is that sugar is addictive, not just because it tastes good or because we like to have more sweetness in our life. To metabolize sugar, the pancreas secretes a hormone called insulin. Insulin allows the cells in the muscles, fat, and liver to absorb glucose in the blood. The glucose serves as energy to these cells or can be converted into fat when needed. Insulin also affects other metabolic processes, such as the breakdown of fat or protein. However, too much insulin can lead to serious health problems. High levels, also known as hyperinsulinemia, have been linked to obesity, heart disease, and cancer. High blood insulin levels also cause your cells to become resistant to the hormone's effects. Once that happens, we're in trouble. When the body has hyper-insulinated, a vicious cycle is set into motion. The sugar cannot be metabolized, so the excess sugar is stored as fat. Thus, we feel tired and hungry and eat more, especially the quick-burning fuel we crave - carbohydrates, aka sugar, and our body then creates more insulin.

Eventually, the cells resist insulin as there is too much of it, and the wheel keeps turning. The body becomes less sensitive to insulin, and the resulting insulin resistance also leads to inflammation. A vicious cycle can result, with more inflammation causing more insulin resistance and vice versa. Most diseases that keep doctors and hospitals so busy: cardiovascular disease, cancer, arthritis, asthma, ulcerative colitis, Crohn's disease, hepatitis, Alzheimer's, and many others are different forms of inflammation. [5] All this to say, sugar intake needs to be taken seriously, but as mentioned earlier, we need carbohydrates in our diet, so what are the healthy sources of carbohydrates, and how much is good for us?

Some advocates of low-carb diets don't differentiate between simple and complex carbohydrates and say sugar is sugar. Refined or simple carbohydrates include sugars and refined grains that have been stripped of all bran, fiber, and nutrients. These include white bread, pizza dough, pasta, pastries, white flour, white rice, sweet desserts, and many breakfast cereals. Complex carbohydrates are found in peas, beans, whole grains, and vegetables. Both simple and complex carbohydrates are turned into glucose (blood sugar) in the body and are used as energy. Most will agree that refined carbohydrates are not good for us, and my personal experience with the effects of these foods on my body-mind confirms that for me. As for complex carbohydrates, there are several different theories out there.

As a vegetarian for most of my adult life, the bulk of my plate was made up of whole grains and vegetables, and my sources of protein were nuts, beans, and some cheese. I also ate eggs for at least half of that time, and fruit was my first food of the day. Philosophy and logic both played a role in my choices. I didn't like the idea of eating animals and had been taught that it was more ecological to use the land to grow grains than grasses

---

[5] https://www.ncbi.nlm.nih.gov/pmc/articles/PMC3992527/
https://www.ncbi.nlm.nih.gov/pmc/articles/PMC3253025/

to feed grazing animals. The macrobiotic diet claims that it is best to eat the food that hangs from trees, like fruit, in the morning, the ground vegetables, like lettuce, kale, cabbage, cucumbers, zucchini, etc., in the midday, and root vegetables in the evening. This also suits my preference to eat light in the morning as mornings are when I have the most energy to exercise, and fruits digest quickly. They also facilitate the evacuation of waste eliminated from our body tissues at night. I also had yogurt or kefir after my fruit in the morning to feed my intestines probiotics. I was reasonably healthy during those years and had no weight issues because I avoided refined or processed foods and rarely added sugar or sugary liquids like honey or maple syrup to my food. Despite this, my diet was still relatively high in sugar intake because I usually added bread or other grains to satisfy my hunger. I was eating to feel full instead of satiated, which is not the same. The resulting excess of carbohydrates and bulk made me feel sluggish after meals and often a little bloated.

The lingering "hunger" I felt after eating was not just because my taste buds had been stimulated or I didn't have enough to eat but was actually a sugar craving. Eating until I felt full had the effect of diminishing my desire to ingest any more food. As I got older, my metabolism slowed down, and the result was that I had less energy and lost some lean muscle mass. I changed my exercise routines to focus more on building muscle tissue and speeding up my metabolism, which helped but with limited success. At some point, I started hearing about low-carb diets that focus on using fat to fuel energy production instead of sugar. I knew that despite adhering to what I thought was a healthy diet and generally avoiding sugary desserts, I was still addicted to sugar, so I began to investigate these alternatives.

The main principle behind low-carb diets is that they shift the body from being a sugar-burning machine to a fat-burning machine. The idea is that sugar is a quicker energy source than fat but not as long-lasting as a fuel source. One could compare sugar burning to burning paper, while fat burning would be like burning a slow-burning log. Decreasing the intake of carbohydrates lowers blood sugar and insulin produced in response to the sugar, setting off a process called ketosis. The body produces ketones when it has limited access to glucose (blood sugar).

When eating a low-carb diet, insulin levels go down, and fatty acids are released from body fat stores in large amounts. Many of these fatty acids are transferred to the liver, where they are oxidized and turned into ketones (or ketone bodies). These molecules can provide energy for the body. Unlike fatty acids, ketones can cross the blood-brain barrier and provide energy for the brain in the absence of glucose. The widely promoted belief that fat is bad for you has been turned upside down by the proponents of low-carb diets. The cause of excess fat and all its associated negative effects is not excess fat but excess sugar. Of course, there are good and bad fats, which is also a controversial subject that I shall not go into here as this is not a nutrition book, but it is important to note that if you consume sugar with fat, even good fats will not be properly metabolized.

There are many diets out there, and as varied as their theories are, they each can sound convincing. My personal experience has taught me to hesitate to advocate a particular diet as I have changed my mind about the "right" diet several times. I believe it is important for each of us to educate ourselves about the physiology of the human body and the science behind each theory and test it with our own bodies to draw our own conclusions. I also believe that our needs are not only different but will vary at different times and in different circumstances for each of us. My purpose here is to share what I believe are basic general principles of wholesome nutrition that most agree on and apply to all of us. Limiting sugar intake is one of the most important, so I have given the subject the attention I believe it deserves.

Eat Whole Foods

Another basic principle is to eat whole foods, in other words, as they are produced by Mother Nature rather than processed or engineered by humans. Simply put, avoid the central aisles in the grocery store that contain the cans and boxes and focus on the fresh produce that is usually close to the outer walls. Don't underestimate the importance of eating organic fruits and vegetables, and if you eat animal sources of protein, eat grass-fed ruminant meats and eggs from pasture-raised chickens. These should be free of hormones and antibiotics and not modified in any other way. In addition to being spared of the toxic effects of food additives, pesticides, and inhumanely treated animals, sustainably cultivated and raised foods are far richer in essential nutrients, so any extra money you spend will save you a lot more in medical and pharmaceutical expenses.

It's Not Just What We Eat but How We Eat

How we cook and eat also affects how well we are fed. We eat our feelings. If you're upset or angry when it's time to prepare a meal, take some time to cool your jets before preparing your meal. It may sound airy-fairy, but energy is real, and your mental-emotional state while preparing and eating the food will affect how you process it. Try not to use too much water when you steam or boil your vegetables not to leech valuable nutrients into the water. Take time to chew your food so it is more thoroughly digested and assimilated. Even if you are cooking for yourself, it's worth it to pay attention to creating a tasty dish that you will enjoy and will be welcomed by the incredible team of organs and microorganisms in your body.

When we eat and how often we eat also plays an important role in how food impacts our health. The first meal of the day is called breakfast because it breaks the fasting period between the evening meal of the previous day and the morning meal. Sleep provides necessary rest for our body and mind. Fasting provides necessary rest for our digestive system and frees up energetic resources for our entire system to regenerate itself.

Apparently, it requires up to 60% of our energy to digest food. The same enzymes that help us digest our food perform many other crucial functions when they are not busy processing our food.

How long we fast between meals is determined by familial and cultural norms, our personal lifestyle and dietary choices, and physiological states. Ten thousand years ago, we were hunter-gatherers in the Paleolithic age before agriculture came along. I would imagine that we would go to sleep not long after dark and wake up when the sun rose. It might be several hours before we could scrounge up enough food to have breakfast, so a good 14-18 hours would pass before putting food into our bellies. How many meals we had on any given day and what we ate or how much we ate would depend on what was available. Then when we discovered how to cultivate plants and animals, and our source of food was more predictable, we could break our fast earlier in the day, and our mealtimes could follow a more regular schedule. Perhaps as labor became more organized, especially with the industrial age, so did mealtime rituals. Mealtimes are also opportunities to commune, so eating together at agreed times was not only a matter of convenience but also to hang out after a morning of hard work or at the end of a day's work. With the advent of artificial lighting with gas and electricity, workdays could extend into the evening hours, and supper could start later and extend longer. All these factors undoubtedly contributed to the popular norm of the breakfast-lunch-supper routine.

Then, in more recent times, many of us enjoy more flexible work schedules, and more free time, which allows for adding snacks to the mix. When we add in the factor of the food industry capitalizing on the addictive effect of high sugar and/or salt content foods like coffee shop pastries, sweet drinks, and other junk foods, the resulting insulin spike makes us want to eat more often. The increasing popularity of low-carb diets and the practice of intermittent fasting (i.e., not eating for 14-18 hours after our evening meal) to reset our hyper-insulated bodies to fat-burning mode is bringing us back to an eating regimen quite like our Paleolithic ancestors, especially if we also choose to eat organic and sustainably cultivated foods. Whether we choose to be vegetarians, vegans, or omnivores, each with their varieties of dietary principles, when it comes to *when* we should eat, there is a phenomenon called **circadian rhythms** that can serve as a reliable guiding principle.

Circadian Rhythms

"Running like clockwork" is an appropriate metaphor to describe a well-tuned body. Just as a car engine will run smoothly when its timing is properly adjusted, our bodies will run more or less smoothly depending on whether we are in sync with the daily waxing and waning of a 24-hour biological cycle called **circadian rhythms.** Circadian rhythms are physical, mental, and behavioral changes that follow a daily cycle. They respond primarily to light and darkness in an organism's environment. Sleeping at night and being awake during the day is an example of a light-related circadian rhythm. Circadian rhythms are found in most living things, including animals, plants, and many tiny microbes.

The study of circadian rhythms is called chronobiology.[6] Our body is equipped with a biological clock, actually many biological clocks, coordinated by a master clock called the SCM (suprachiasmatic nucleus) in the central part of our brain called the hypothalamus that serves as an innate timing device to regulate all our body functions. It receives direct input from the eyes. The main cue influencing circadian rhythms is daylight. This light can turn genes that control the molecular structure of biological clocks on or off. Changing the light-dark cycles can speed up, slow down, or reset biological clocks and circadian rhythms. Circadian rhythms can influence sleep-wake cycles, hormone release, eating habits and digestion, body temperature, and other important bodily functions. Biological clocks that run fast or slow can result in disrupted or abnormal circadian rhythms. Irregular rhythms have been linked to various chronic health conditions, such as sleep disorders, obesity, diabetes, depression, bipolar disorder, and seasonal affective disorder. Circadian rhythms help determine our sleep patterns. The body's master clock, or SCN, controls the production of melatonin, a hormone that makes you sleepy. It receives information about incoming light from the optic nerves, which relay information from the eyes to the brain. When there is less light—like at night—the SCN tells the brain to make more melatonin, so you get drowsy.

---

[6] https://www.nigms.nih.gov/education/fact-sheets/Pages/circadian-rhythms.aspx

The ancient healing art of Ayurveda calls the practice of attuning our bodies to the circadian rhythms *Dinacharya*, from the Sanskrit word made up of *dina*, meaning day, and *acharya*, meaning activity. So, *Dinacharya* is a daily routine designed to maintain and connect us to our circadian rhythms or internal body clocks. Ayurveda tells us that on any given day, there are two cycles of change that exist—the sun cycle and the moon cycle—and they're connected with the ayurvedic body type, or doshic constitution: *Vata* (space and air), *Pitta* (fire and water), or *Kapha* (earth and water). [7] Dividing our day into six 4-hour segments, 10 pm to 2 am and 10am to 2pm are considered Pitta times of the day; 2 am to 6 am and 2 pm to 6 pm are considered Vata times of the day; and 6 am to10 am and 6 pm to10 pm are considered Kapha times of the day. Though I have generally followed these energetic cycles for many years regarding my eating, sleeping, and activity times, I am not sufficiently knowledgeable in Ayurveda to interpret the complexity of how the doshas, and circadian rhythms interact. However, I was able to find an excellent description online simply and clearly articulated by a yogi named Ashley Josephine Zuberi: "Pitta is the energy of transformation and of metabolism. The fire in Pitta corresponds directly with our ability to digest food and extract the nutrients from our food to transform our bodies."

If you have a Pitta deficiency, your digestion is probably weak. During the (fiery) Pitta times of the day,

---

[7] https://www.artofliving.org/ayurveda-dinacharya-use-circadian-rhythm-your-body-optimal-wellness

your digestive power is at its greatest. This is why in Ayurveda (and many cultures, for that matter), the largest meal of the day is eaten at mid-day between that 10 am to 2pm timeframe when we're best able to digest heavy meals. When you look at when most Americans eat their largest and heaviest meal of the day, it's right in that (muddy) Kapha timeframe when our digestion is slowest. You might argue that the body goes back into Pitta time in the evening, so it shouldn't matter how large a meal we eat at night, but food isn't the only thing the body has to digest. In the evening Pitta time, the body starts to digest mental energy, and the body's repair mechanisms turn on as we sleep. That is why in Ayurveda, it's best to be in bed and resting from 10 pm to 2 am so that the body can have the time to do all this transforming and metabolizing on the inside. Plus, that fire needs a chance to rest, lest we burn out.

Have you ever had difficulty getting out of bed in the morning, even when you think you're getting enough sleep? Well, in Ayurveda, when you look at the times of day, you'll see that once we hit 6 am, we're in a Kapha time of day—the slowest, groggiest, and hardest time of the day to get motivated! In Ayurveda, it's recommended to rise before the sun, which is often right around that 6 am mark (Daylight Savings Time ruined the natural cycles, so we must consider that now). In Arizona, where they don't recognize Daylight Savings Time, the sun rises around 5:30 am. Getting up around this time ensures you're getting up before the Kapha time hits, and for most people, depending on what time they went to sleep and their doshic constitution, they'll amazingly find that waking up before 6 am is easier than they imagined.

Have you ever woken up in the middle of the night between 2 to 6 am? Perhaps your mind was running wild with ideas, or you were worried about something coming up at work. This is representative of Vata, which primarily resides in the mind. When we look at Western medical science and the stages of sleep, it's during those last stages of sleep (REM sleep) that we get the craziest dreams. We know from research that if we get up before our sleep stages are complete, we'll most likely not feel energized upon waking.

Vata energy also corresponds with creativity and cognitive ability. This is why the afternoon period between 2 pm to 6 pm is a great time for brainstorming and creative projects. It's also the best time to meditate because we're better able to access and control our mental abilities. If you get up before 6 am and meditate, which Ayurveda recommends, you've set yourself up for a successful day.

Finally, Kapha energy is the slowest and needs the most motivation. From 6 am to 10 am, when we're getting ready for our day, it's a great time to work out and get the stimulation that your body needs to move throughout the rest of the day with ease and energy. In the evening, it's a good time to start to slow down and get ready for bed.

You can see that each time span honors one of the two aspects of each doshic quality. In the evening, Pitta needs to calm down, but in the middle of the day, Pitta energy is at its highest, which can be an intense time. Kapha energy needs to be stimulated in the morning, but in the evening, the slow and peaceful qualities need to be honored. And for Vata, the morning is about resting, and the afternoon is about using that mental energy in a focused and efficient manner. When you overlay the doshas with time, space, and personal constitution, the puzzle pieces of balance start to all fall in place.[8]

In accordance with our biological clock, the yogic teachings advise us not to eat a large breakfast or even skip it if we practice intermittent fasting as I do (more about that coming up) and make our midday meal the larger meal. We are also advised to eat more lightly in the evening and to be done eating by 7 pm so that our meal is mostly digested by the time we hit the sack, which should be by 9 or 10 latest, allowing for seasonal variations of daylight time. It is best to rise by 5 or 5:30 am before the sun rises. This will allow us 7 to 8 hours of sleep. It is not just how much we sleep but when we sleep that ensures that our body is well-rested and regenerated. Sleep quality is crucial for our physical and mental health, so this will be dealt with in more depth in a later section.

Intermittent Fasting

Fasting is one of the world's most ancient and widespread healing traditions. Hippocrates (c 460 – c370 BC) prescribed and championed the practice of fasting. He

---

[8] http://ashleyjosephine.com/ayurveda-circadian-rhythm/

wrote, "To eat when you are sick is to feed your illness." It has been used not only for weight loss but to improve concentration, extend life, prevent Alzheimer's, prevent insulin resistance, and even reverse the entire aging process. There are, of course, many ways to fast, and not all of them are good for you. People who are brittle diabetics, those with a history of eating disorders like anorexia and bulimia, and pregnant or breastfeeding women should not attempt fasting unless under they are under the close supervision of a doctor.[9] I have experimented with different variations of fasting and the one that I consider to be the most sustainable and safe is intermittent fasting. Intermittent fasting is an eating pattern where you cycle between periods of eating and fasting.

There are several variations of intermittent fasting, but the most effective is the 16:8 method, which involves fasting for 16 hours from the end of the day's last meal to the following day's first meal and restricting the period of eating to the 8 hours between fasts. Some of the changes that occur in your body during fasting include: the insulin levels in your blood drop, which facilitates fat-burning; blood levels of growth hormone may increase, facilitating fat-burning and muscle gain; the body induces important cellular repair processes, such as removing waste from cells; and beneficial changes in

---

[9] https://healthblog.uofmhealth.org/wellness-prevention/intermittent-fasting-it-right-for-you#:~:text=Besides%20weight%20loss%2C%20are%20there,motor%20coordination%20and%20improved%20sleep.

several genes and molecules related to longevity and protection against disease.

Weight loss is another benefit. Lower insulin levels, higher growth hormone levels, and increased amounts of norepinephrine (noradrenaline) all increase the breakdown of body fat and facilitate its use for energy. For this reason, short-term fasting increases your metabolic rate by 3.6-14%, helping you burn even more calories. Intermittent fasting works on both sides of the calorie equation. It boosts your metabolic rate (increases calories out) and reduces the amount of food you eat (reduces calories in).

Intermittent fasting has been shown to have major benefits for insulin resistance and lead to an impressive reduction in blood sugar levels. This implies that intermittent fasting may be highly protective for people at risk of developing type 2 diabetes.

Several studies show that intermittent fasting may enhance the body's resistance to oxidative stress and help fight inflammation, another key driver of all sorts of common diseases. Studies also show that intermittent fasting can improve numerous risk factors for heart disease, such as blood pressure, cholesterol levels, triglycerides, and inflammatory markers though most of these studies are animal studies and have yet to be proven in humans. Intermittent fasting has also been shown to help prevent cancer in animal studies. One paper showed that it could reduce side effects caused by chemotherapy in humans. Intermittent fasting may have important benefits for brain health. It may increase the growth of new neurons and protect the brain from damage, and it may also be protective against neurodegenerative diseases like Alzheimer's disease.

Intermittent fasting has become very popular among the anti-aging crowd. Given the known benefits for metabolism and all sorts of health markers, it makes sense that intermittent fasting could help you live a longer and healthier life.[10]

A growing body of research suggests that the timing of the fast is key. "We have evolved to be in sync with the day/night cycle, i.e., a circadian rhythm. Our metabolism has adapted to daytime food and nighttime sleep. Nighttime eating is well associated with a higher risk of obesity, as well as diabetes. Based on this, researchers from the University of Alabama conducted a study with a small group of obese men with pre-diabetes. They compared a form of intermittent fasting called 'early time-restricted feeding,' where all meals were fit into an early eight-hour period of the day (7 am to 3 pm) or spread out over 12 hours (between 7 am and 7 pm). Both groups maintained their weight (did not gain or lose), but after five weeks, the eight-hour group had dramatically lower insulin levels and significantly improved insulin sensitivity, as well as significantly lower blood pressure. The best part? The eight-hour group also had significantly decreased appetite. They weren't starving. Just changing the timing of meals, by eating earlier in the day and extending the overnight

---

[10] https://www.healthline.com/nutrition/10-health-benefits-of-intermittent-fasting#section10

fast, significantly benefited metabolism even in people who didn't lose a single pound."[11]

Move Your Body

Life is always on the move. What appears to be still is only relatively still as even elements that appear to be inert are composed of atoms that are always on the move and can react if subjected to enough energy. As long as we are alive, our bodies vibrate with life energy. All five of our senses require movement to function. Try focusing your eyes on the tip of a pencil and watch it disappear when your eyes stop moving. Your ear hears sounds because the vibration of the sound vibrates the ear drum connected to the brain through tiny nerves that transmit these sensations to the brain. Your nose smells because the olfactory neurons in our nose are stimulated by odor particles moving in the air, which send that message to the brain through their neural pathways. When we taste, the sensory receptors in the taste buds on our tongue send a message to our brain. Like water that becomes stagnant when it stays still for too long, our body's systems will stagnate and crystallize if energy isn't circulating. The typical lifestyle of people in developed countries does not support the essential need for us to move our bodies and align our bodies in such a way that energy can circulate in our bodies. Most of us spend a major part of our day sitting in chairs which, according to Dr. James A. Levine, director of the Mayo Clinic Arizona State University Obesity Solutions

---

[11] https://www.health.harvard.edu/blog/intermittent-fasting-surprising-update-2018062914156

Initiative, kills more people than smoking. According to Dr. Levine and other researchers in the field, "sitting for as little as two continuous hours increases the risk of heart disease, diabetes, metabolic syndrome, cancer, back and neck pain, and other orthopedic problems. Sitting will shorten your life, just like smoking." [12] Even maintaining a regular fitness regimen cannot counteract the accumulated effects of sitting 8 to 12 hours a day between exercise sessions!

Dr. Levine claims that going to the gym for 30 minutes a day does not reverse the effects and tops off the miserable news with the claim that for every hour we sit, we lose two hours of life expectancy. Sitting is now considered the new smoking as it increases your rate of lung cancer by over 50 percent. The good news is that exercise and even just moving the body mitigate the negative effects of sitting, and it is not that difficult to develop the habit of standing at your computer rather than sitting in a chair, which removes most of the harmful effects of chairs even though there is not much movement going on when we stand. Standing desks are widely available now, some even with treadmills, and I shall share my economical homemade version in a later section of this book. However, I first want to share the amazing benefits of exercise in general, the particular benefits of different types of exercise, and the importance of including more than one type of exercise in your weekly routine.

---

[12] *Get Up: Why Your Chair Is Killing You and What You Can Do About It.* James A. Levine StMartin's Publishing; July 2014

The application of specific exercises in accord with a more natural lifestyle and that support functionality and physical and mental health does not require any great expense of time, money, or equipment. You can get extremely fit in just a few hours a week if you have a balance of extensive low-intensity movement, periodic high-intensity, short-duration strength training sessions, and occasional all-out sprints. The kind of fitness I am referring to optimizes your capacity to perform a broad range of skills and activities involving strength, power, speed, and endurance with a high power-to-weight ratio.

You will get the best results if you vary your routines, align your workout choices with your energy level and motivation, pursue fun and inspiring goals, and ensure you allow sufficient recovery. Frequent long and strenuous workouts are inefficient for weight loss, lean muscle building, or general health. Wholesome and natural eating habits (respecting circadian rhythms, eating foods offered to us by Mother Nature rather than processed by the food industry, and educating ourselves to know more about nutrition) combined with frequent low-intensity exercise and occasional brief and intense strength and sprint sessions will stimulate your metabolic rate to burn fat and build lean muscle.

Yoga

The term *yoga* is popularly used to refer to an ancient system of posture sequences performed with attention to one's breath and proper alignment. Actually, this more physical aspect of yoga is just one of eight branches of yoga practice. In Sanskrit, the word *yoga* translates literally as yoke and refers to the joining of body, mind, and spirit. The eight branches of yoga cover various disciplines of body-mind training and lifestyle designed to facilitate this integration process. The first two, the *yamas* and *nyamas*, describe the five things not to do and the five things to do as the foundation of a yogic lifestyle—basically a kind of moral code like the Ten Commandments. The third branch or limb of the yoga tree is *asana,* which translates literally as seat, and refers to the posture sequences commonly referred to as yoga.

The meaning of seat here is not restricted to the act of sitting but rather cultivating stability of body and mind, whether in movement or relative stillness. Perhaps the ultimate expression of asana is *padmasana* or lotus posture, the cross-legged posture adopted for sitting in meditation. The fourth limb is *pranayama,* which is the practice of mastering the energy of the body through breath control techniques. The fifth limb is *pratyahara,* which is the practice of reeling in the senses to focus on their source within rather than the external objects they are perceiving. *Dharana,* or one-pointed concentration, is the sixth limb, and *dhyana*, or meditation, is the seventh. Finally, the eighth limb is *samadhi*, or oneness, which can be experienced as a temporary conditional state while one still has an ego or as a permanent unconditional transcendence of the ego state. This book touches upon all these aspects of the yogic lifestyle. This section on exercise will focus on the benefits of Hatha Yoga.

Hatha yoga is the term used today to describe the practice of asana yoga; the series of physical postures combined with breath control. The original Hatha yoga was practiced by Hindu and Tibetan Buddhist yogis of the Vajrayana school as a transformative tantric practice. In Sanskrit, the word *hatha* means force; *ha* means sun, and *tha* means moon. Body postures, breath, and mind control were used as a means to preserve vital energy in the head (the "moon") from dripping down the central channel and being burned by the fire (the "sun") at the perineum.

Mastering these techniques requires qualified guidance and years of practice in body-mind-breath control referred to in the eight branches of yoga described earlier. Today, the term Hatha yoga is attributed to the more accessible practice of physical postures in conjunction with mindfulness and control of the breath. What can be confusing is that it is now often contrasted with speedier and more exertive posture flows called Vinyasa, of which the main school is called Ashtanga. A popular and respected yogi named Patabhi Jois appropriated the name for his system of posture flow sequences, which, properly speaking, is just another version of Hatha yoga that is part of the third limb of Ashtanga called *asana*.

Benefits of Hatha Yoga

The virtues of practicing yoga have been extolled over thousands of years. The practice of Hatha yoga, in particular, has produced a wide range of benefits depending on the poses practiced, the intensity (calculated by awareness, not sweat), and the length and frequency of practice. Modern scientists confirm these benefits for general health and well-being and therapy for certain medical conditions. Documented benefits stemming from practicing Hatha yoga postures, breathing, and meditation include:

General Benefits

- Relieves fatigue and increases energy
- Stimulates the immune system
- Reduces stress
- Improves concentration and frame of mind

Musculoskeletal Benefits

- Decompresses and lengthens the spine, relieves lower backache, and counters the effects of aging on the spine and bones
- Helps to correct posture
- Relieves sciatic and arthritis pain and can slow down the progress of arthritis
- Keeps muscles flexible, joints movable
- Helps to tone and strengthen muscles

Cardiovascular Benefits

- Can help to stabilize blood pressure

- Improves circulation

Respiratory Benefits

- Can improve breathing capacity and, in some cases, asthmatic symptoms

- Increases the elasticity of lung tissue

Digestive Benefits

- Rejuvenates abdominal organs and improves digestion

One or several of these benefits may motivate one to take up this practice, but the greatest benefit of yoga, which means Oneness, Unity, or Wholeness, is the dissolving of the sense of separation from others and the world around us, and especially within oneself, which is the root from which all conflict and disease stem.

I like to vary the types of exercise I do to focus on different aspects of physical fitness, which I shall describe in this chapter, but I include several hours of Hatha yoga each week as it is an excellent foundation for all forms of exercise. For example, the flexibility gained from the stretching postures in yoga serves me in strength workouts as the increased range of motion allows more force to be generated in the movement. I am not referring to passive stretching just before a workout, which is quite popular yet not generally recommended, but the dynamic stretching involved in most of the yoga postures and movements (contracting combined with lengthening), which more effectively lengthens muscles. Additionally, the space created in the joints of the body in most yoga postures removes resistance to allow more freedom of movement for all activities. The more passive stretches used in restorative yoga styles benefit us as well because they teach the body-mind how to let go of unconscious holding to allow energy or life force to circulate more freely. Besides the musculoskeletal and respiratory benefits, I have also found that many of the movements are used in other forms of exercise, sports, martial arts, and dance. For example, when I took up surfing a few years ago, I was impressed by how many of the movements involved are movements used in yoga, and many surfers also practice yoga to inform and support their performance and prevent injuries.

Complementary Fitness Exercises

For many years, my exercise mainly consisted of what today would be called restorative yoga and occasional jogging, swimming, and walking. It kept me reasonably fit, but when I was introduced to some more intense Vinyasa yoga styles involving speedier movements and strengthening postures, I enjoyed more vitality. It is antithetical to the spirit of yoga to practice it competitively or for the sake of accomplishing a more challenging posture, but I got a little hooked into that mindset for a while and found that I was getting injured more often and began to look for alternate forms of exercise to strengthen and inform my postures. This eventually led to researching a complete physical fitness program incorporating aerobic fitness, strength training, core exercises, balance training, flexibility, and some stretching. It isn't necessary to fit all these elements into every fitness session but factoring them into your weekly exercise schedule can help you promote fitness for life. Advanced yogis with more rigorous practices will get most of these benefits without needing to include alternate forms of exercise like the ones I shall mention below; however, I highly recommend that you do as much of your exercise outdoors as possible to benefit from the vital energy circulating freely in the ambient air (preferably not too polluted). I also feel it is important to include movements that inform and support activities we may need to use in our various life activities, such as walking, running, climbing, lifting, etc.

HIIT

HIIT, or High-Intensity Interval Training, is a form of interval training, a cardiovascular exercise strategy alternating short periods of intense anaerobic exercise with less intense recovery periods until near exhaustion. There are many variations, but these intense workouts typically last under 30 minutes, with times varying based on a participant's current fitness level and the session's intensity. There are many different systems of interval durations. I like to use the Tabata system of 20 seconds of ultra-intense exercise followed by 10 seconds of rest, repeated continuously for 4 minutes (8 cycles), with a minute rest between cycles. So, for a 30-minute workout, I choose 6 different exercises (usually bodyweight only) repeated 8 times each. However, I like to change it up from time to time, so I also practice other variations. For my weekly cardio session, I do sprint intervals.

HIIT workouts improve athletic capacity and condition and improve glucose metabolism.[13] Research has shown that HIIT regimens produce significant reductions in the fat mass of the whole body.[14] It takes a certain degree of motivation to exercise at this intensity. Still, both the effort intervals and the overall duration of the exercise (as low as 10 minutes and no higher than 30 minutes) are relatively short, so I am more motivated to do a 20-minute series of sprint intervals, for example of 20 seconds each with 40 second walks in between, than to run continuously at a moderate pace for 30- 60 minutes. The bonus is that it gives you more bang for your buck as your metabolism is stimulated not only while you perform the workout. You are burning fat and getting energy from the process that primarily metabolizes protein and healthy fat. The combination of fasting to lower the blood sugar and insulin levels and the stimulation of growth hormone enables your body to switch from being

---

[13] Laursen PB, Jenkins DG (2002). "The Scientific Basis for High-Intensity Interval Training." *Sports Medicine* (Review). **32** (1): 53–73.

[14] Zhang, Haifeng; Tong, Tom K.; Qiu, Weifeng; Zhang, Xu; Zhou, Shi; Liu, Yang; He, Yuxiu (2017-01-01). "Comparable Effects of High-Intensity Interval Training and Prolonged Continuous Exercise Training on Abdominal Visceral Fat Reduction in Obese Young Women". *Journal of Diabetes Research*. **2017**: 5071740.

a sugar-burning machine to a fat-burning machine, which leads to losing fat and gaining muscle.

I like to exercise in the morning during my fasting period as I am not using energy to digest at that time, and the stimulation of endorphins and other growth hormones not only gives me a boost of energy but also suppresses my appetite. One can get a similar effect from a cup of coffee, but this effect is not sustained when one has caffeine regularly as the artificial stimulation of adrenalin eventually flips into a drop of energy and the craving for another cup of brew. So, when I feel like I could use a little boost to motivate me before my morning workout, I get more sustained energy from a cup of decaffeinated coffee with MCT coconut oil, and it's delicious.

Cardio

Cardio fitness is short for cardiovascular and cardiorespiratory fitness. Cardiovascular refers to the ability of your heart and blood vessels to transport blood during a workout. Cardiovascular endurance improves heart health and reduces your chances of experiencing heart disease. Cardiorespiratory endurance can be defined as the ability of your heart, lungs, and muscles to work together over a long stretch of time. Functionally, cardiovascular endurance benefits and those of cardiorespiratory endurance are essentially the same, so cardio refers to both. Cardio is what most people refer to when they are talking about "aerobic exercise." Aerobic exercise is any exercise that uses oxygen, and cardio refers to your heart pumping. So, when you do a cardio workout, you *are* working aerobically. Examples include running, cycling, swimming, rowing, and even long walks or climbs.

Cardio can include weighted activities too, but it's usually done circuit-style to increase your heart rate over a longer period of time rather than lifting weights to increase strength, power, or muscle mass. Conversely, anaerobic exercise refers to exercise without using oxygen. The high-intensity exercises such as HIIT described earlier, and any exercise that requires short bursts of energy, like lifting weights to improve strength, sprinting short distances, or jumping, are examples of anaerobic exercise. Cardio/aerobic exercise will help you burn energy while performing the activity because your body is continually fueled by oxygen. Whereas in anaerobic activities, your body cannot get enough oxygen when doing the intense short burst exercises, so it needs to burn fat to fuel its activity, which helps you to continue burning the fat fuel for several hours after the activity. A complete fitness strategy should include both cardio/aerobic and anaerobic exercise. How much you do of each depends on your goals or needs. If your goal is to be a long-distance runner, swimmer, or preparing for a Himalayan trek, then you will be dedicating a greater proportion of time to aerobic exercise than anaerobic exercise. You will benefit from more anaerobic workouts if you're training for any sport that requires a lot of short-burst energy output for fast movements like hockey, sprints, tennis, or even weightlifting. There are, of course, sports that involve both aerobic endurance and anaerobic fitness, like soccer, climbing, tennis, and many others, which would require both types of exercise. For specific health goals, there are also a variety of approaches.

For example, if weight loss is your goal, then either aerobic or anaerobic exercise can support you. Aerobic exercise will be your way to burn fat if you have more affinity for moderate exercise over a long period of time. If you prefer shorter periods of intense exercise, your hard work will be rewarded by spending less time doing your workout yet burning fat for hours after. Some forms of exercise, like swimming, Hatha yoga, and even surfing, will be aerobic or anaerobic, depending on how you are doing them. For example, when I trained on my high school swim team, I was swimming at anaerobic intensity a lot of the time, whereas my long-distance swims in more recent years were aerobic activities. When I started practicing Hatha yoga for therapeutic reasons, I was efforting at a more moderate level, whereas the Vinyasa styles of yoga I practiced later in life that required quicker transitions between poses and more strength provided some anaerobic benefits. Level of proficiency is also a factor in the equation. I am not an advanced surfer, so I don't have the skills (yet!) to move quickly and get long rides, as I am not exerting myself at the same level as a seasoned surfer. At different periods in your life, factors like a slower metabolism, lower energy level, muscle atrophy, joints compromised by inflammation or deterioration, or scarring from previous injuries will also influence your choice of types of exercise.

When I found that my metabolism was slowing down and I was losing some muscle mass and feeling tired more often as I got older, I supplemented my regular moderate Hatha yoga practice and occasional jogging with more intense anaerobic exercise. I began alternating between whole-body HIIT workouts, strength workouts, and weekly sprinting workouts combined with a cardio warmup jog. I also found that short, intense runs were kinder to my slightly compromised knee joints than moderately paced long-distance runs. So, at my fitness level, what works for me is 2 or 3 HIIT and strength workouts per week, one cardio (aerobic and anaerobic) session per week (mine is a 10-minute jogging warmup followed by 10 to 20 minutes of sprint intervals), and some Hatha yoga sessions, playful movement, and walking and biking in between. It might sound like a lot for some of you, but it works out to only an hour or two per day.

Strength

Strength training, also known as weight or resistance training, is physical activity designed to improve muscular fitness by exercising a specific muscle or muscle group against external resistance, including free weights, weight machines, or your own body weight. The basic principle is to apply a load and overload the muscle so that it adapts and gets stronger. Strength training is not just about bodybuilders lifting weights in a gym. Regular strength or resistance training also helps prevent the natural loss of lean muscle mass that comes with aging.

While building up muscle mass may elevate your body-image, many more benefits exist.

- **Develop strong bones.** Strength training can increase bone density and reduce the risk of osteoporosis by stressing your bones.

- **Manage your weight.** Strength training can help you manage or lose weight and increase your metabolism to help you burn more calories. Post-exercise oxygen consumption (EPOC)—the calories your body continues to burn after a workout—keeps your metabolism active after exercising, much longer than after an aerobic workout.

- **Enhance your quality of life.** Strength training may enhance your quality of life and improve your ability to do everyday activities. Building muscle can also contribute to better balance and may reduce your risk of falling. This can help you maintain independence as you age.

- **Manage chronic conditions.** Strength training can reduce the signs and symptoms of many chronic conditions, such as arthritis, back pain, obesity, heart disease, depression, and diabetes.

- **Sharpen your thinking skills.** Some research suggests that regular strength training and aerobic exercise may help improve thinking and learning skills for older adults.

Rest one full day between exercising each specific muscle group to give your muscles time to recover. Also, be careful to listen to your body. If a strength training exercise causes pain, stop the exercise. Consider trying a lower weight or trying it again in a few days.

It's important to use proper technique in strength training to avoid injuries. If you're new to weight training, work with a trainer or fitness specialist to learn the correct form and technique. Remember to breathe as you strength train. You don't need to spend hours a day lifting weights to benefit from strength training. You can see significant improvement in your strength with just two or three 20- or 30-minute weight training sessions per week.

Natural Exercise

There are many more ways to move our bodies and get exercise than the types of exercise I have described, each providing particular benefits to body and mind and the quality of our life in general. These include individual and team sports, martial arts practiced solo or sparring with a partner, dancing solo or with a partner or group, climbing, hiking, trekking, biking and walking rather than driving or taking a bus are all beneficial.

There is also *natural exercise*. For primal humans, that meant lots of walking, lifting and carrying things, pushing things, pulling themselves up, climbing, crawling on all fours to creep up on prey, frequent intervals of sprinting to run after or run away from wild animals, and lots of squatting to rest, eat, and evacuate. They didn't sit in chairs for long periods or spend hours at a gym running on treadmills or plugging themselves into machines designed to target and beef up specific muscles. Their exercises were functional, i.e., meeting the requirements of their lifestyle. While it is true that our "civilized" life today does not require most of us to hunt, run from wild animals, or even walk to our destinations, this comfortable and convenient lifestyle has had the unfortunate effect of compromising our health, not to mention the environment that is essential to our well-being. In particular, while offering many advantages, the digital age has undermined our physical and mental health. Most of us know that electromagnetic radiation from our cellphones, computers, and other telecommunication devices are damaging the cells of our body and brains, causing cancer, and sapping our energy, not to mention compromising our psycho-social sensitivity and skills. Still, unfortunately, most of us are not about to change our habits. Also, as mentioned earlier, recent research has revealed that sitting is just as bad, if not worse, than the radiation emitted by the screens of our devices!

Play

A final thought about exercise: It doesn't have to be a "workout" in a gym or even *work*! I have experienced some functional fitness sessions that felt more like play than work, even though they are based on lots of bio-mechanical knowledge and experience. I once met a man who was very fit on the beach where I live. I had seen him around quite often but never in any of the local yoga or other exercise classes I attended in the area. I asked him what type of exercise he practiced, and he told me that he goes to the beach or into the jungle and plays with objects around him, like jumping over fallen trees, balancing by walking along a log, lifting heavy rocks, running on the beach, or swimming in the ocean. Admittedly I haven't explored this form of natural and playful movement, but I was impressed. Soon after, I discovered a playful form of exercise that uses primal, animalistic movements, also close to my home in Costa Rica. It is called Movenplay, and it consists of sessions designed by Alex Herrera, a former tennis pro and experienced martial arts adept who creates playful choreographies of movement that are accessible to a wide range of fitness and coordination levels, are lots of fun, and teach both the body and mind to become more agile. While the overall experience is playful and exhilarating, it also demands one's full attention to coordinate one's own movements and interactive movements with other participants. One could call this conscious playing. Alex often reminds his students to "play for keeps."

5
Sleep

Sleep is as important to your health and well-being as good nutrition and exercise. Lack of sleep will not just make you cranky for an hour or two after you get up. The cumulative effect of sleep deprivation can seriously impact both physical and mental health and your capacity to function and relate to others from day to day.

Cardiovascular Health

While you sleep, your blood pressure goes down, giving your heart and blood vessels a rest. The less sleep you get, the longer your blood pressure stays up during a 24-hour cycle. High blood pressure can lead to heart disease, including stroke.[15]

Weight Management

Several factors link sleep deprivation to weight gain. During the deep, slow-wave part of your sleep cycle, the amount of glucose in your blood drops. Not enough time

---

[15] https://www.webmd.com/sleep-disorders/benefits-sleep-more

in this deepest stage means you don't get that break to allow a reset—like leaving the volume turned up. Your body will have a harder time responding to your cells' needs and blood sugar levels. By allowing yourself to reach and remain in this deep sleep, you're less likely to get type 2 diabetes.[16] Higher glucose levels also lead to putting on pounds of fat. Furthermore, when you're well-rested, you're less hungry. Being sleep-deprived messes with the hormones in your brain— leptin and ghrelin—that control appetite. With those out of balance, your resistance to the temptation of unhealthy foods goes down. And when you're tired, you're less likely to want to get up and move your body. Together, it's a recipe for putting on pounds. The time you spend in bed goes hand-in-hand with the time you spend at the table and at the gym to help you manage your weight.[17]

Immunity

Your immune system identifies harmful bacteria and viruses in your body and destroys them to help you ward off illnesses. An ongoing lack of sleep changes the way your immune cells work. They may not attack as quickly, and you could get sick more often. Good nightly rest now can help you avoid that tired, worn-out feeling, as well as spending days in bed as your body tries to recover.[18]

---

[16] https://www.webmd.com/sleep-disorders/benefits-sleep-more
[17] https://www.webmd.com/sleep-disorders/benefits-sleep-more
[18] https://www.webmd.com/sleep-disorders/benefits-sleep-more

Athletic Performance

A good night's sleep is crucial for athletic performance. If your sport requires quick bursts of energy, like wrestling or weightlifting, sleep loss may not affect you as much as endurance sports like running, swimming, and biking. However, insufficient quality sleep robs you of energy and time for muscle repair, and lack of sleep saps your motivation, which is what gets you to the finish line. You'll face a harder mental and physical challenge and see slower reaction times. Proper rest sets you up for your best performance.[19]

Mental Performance

You'll have more trouble retaining and remembering details when you're running low on sleep. Sleep plays a big part in both learning and memory. Insufficient sleep makes it hard to focus and absorb new information, and your brain also doesn't have enough time to store memories properly to pull them up later. Sleep lets your brain catch up so you're ready for what's next.

Your Mood

While you sleep, your brain processes your emotions. Your mind needs this time to recognize and react the right way. When you cut that short, you tend to have more negative emotional reactions and fewer positive ones.

---

[19] https://www.webmd.com/sleep-disorders/benefits-sleep-more

Chronic lack of sleep can also raise the chance of having a mood disorder. One large study showed that when you have insomnia, you're five times more likely to develop depression, and your odds of anxiety or panic disorders are even greater.[20]

How Much Sleep Is Enough?

According to the National Sleep Foundation[21], the amount of sleep we need varies in accordance with our age.

Younger children need much more sleep, and many will need naps to reach their goals. For example, a newborn will need 14-17 hours of sleep, while someone over the age of 65 will need 7-8 hours. These averages reflect the influence of developmental stages on our body's need for sleep. However, individual lifestyles ultimately make for significant differences in how much sleep each of us needs.

Getting the Most Out of Your Sleep

The higher the quality of our sleep, the less we need. The following habits will help you get more out of your sleep:

- maintaining a regular sleep/wake schedule

---

[20] Neckelmann, D. et al., Chronic Insomnia as a Risk Factor for Developing Anxiety and Depression, Sleep. 2007; 30 (7): 873-880.
[21] https://www.sciencedirect.com/science/article/abs/pii/S2352721815000157

- avoiding caffeine, alcohol, nicotine, and other chemicals that interfere with sleep

- making your bedroom a comfortable sleep environment

- establishing a calming pre-sleep routine

- going to sleep when you're truly tired

- not watching the clock at night

- using light to your advantage by exposing yourself to light during the day and limiting light exposure in the evening

- not napping too close to your regular bedtime

- eating and drinking enough—but not too much or too soon before bedtime

- exercising regularly—but not too soon before bedtime

Perhaps the most important factor in ensuring a high quality of sleep is *when* you sleep. As mentioned earlier in this book, we will get more out of our sleep if we respect the biological connection with circadian rhythms. Here is a brief description of the physiology involved in this connection.

As soon as you head to the coffee shop to begin your day, your body is already preparing for sleep. While awake, your body produces a chemical called adenosine that adds up consistently throughout the day and eventually causes drowsiness, signaling that you're ready for bed. Your sleep and its daily relationship with wakefulness are controlled by two systems: your biological clock (or circadian rhythm) and your sleep drive. Your circadian rhythm is the biochemical cycle that repeats roughly every 24 hours and governs sleep, wake time, hunger, body temperature, hormone release, and other subtle rhythms that mesh with the 24-hour day. Your sleep drive (the need for sleep) dictates the amount and intensity of sleep you need based on how long you've been awake. Think of your sleep drive like hunger; it builds throughout the day until it is satisfied.

Practically speaking, we are meant to be active during daylight hours and sleep when it is dark. In accordance with the circadian rhythms, we should be hitting the sack within a few hours after the sun sets, think between 8 pm and 10 pm, depending on the time of year and your latitudinal position on the planet. Where I live in Costa Rica, we are very close to the equator, so there is minimal variation in the daylight hours. The sun always sets at about 5:45 pm and rises around 5:45 am. It is also a small community interspersed in natural surroundings, so it is not lit up at night like big cities. Everyone spends most of their time outside because of the comfortable year-round temperatures, in contrast to many places where people spend a lot more time indoors with artificial lighting, heating, or cooling.

Consequently, most people here are ready to go to bed between 8 pm and 10 pm and rise naturally (no alarm clock) between 5 am and 7 am. However, I have found that I naturally tend to keep the same hours even when I return to Montreal in the summer, where it doesn't get dark until 8 pm or 9 pm. This is because my body is habituated to this schedule, and I wake up naturally when the dawn is just beginning to break. It is also because this schedule leaves me feeling most energetic and productive in the morning, and I feel more rested than when I get the same amount of sleep going to bed later.

6
Self-knowledge

We are both absolute and relative beings. From the point of view of the vision of Oneness, our essential Self is absolute and all-encompassing. It knows no separation in time or space. It will never die because it was never born. It always IS. It knows no separation between self and other. It holds no position of preference, no identity to be attached to. As such, it is not identifiable or definable. Buddhists call it Buddha-nature, and practices such as meditation are tools we use to pierce the veil of illusion that keeps us in the trance of ego, individuality, or separate existence. Buddha means "awake." The ultimate goal of Buddhist practice is to "wake up" from the illusion of separateness to the realization of our True Self.

As described earlier in this book, I experienced a kind of existential crisis in my teen years in which I was confronted with the painful awareness of the ignorance of my origin and destiny while simultaneously knowing that I have no beginning or end. What made it painful was the apparent contradiction between this inner knowing and the thoroughly entrenched belief that my life began when

I was plopped into this world as a baby and will end when my body dies. At the time, I didn't know about meditation or any other technique that could allow me to "think out of the box," i.e., witness and transcend my surface-level-thinking mind and help me resolve the apparent contradiction of my existence. I read some books about the potentials of the human mind and later took some psychology and philosophy courses in university that gave me some perspective on how the mind works, but this conceptual knowledge did not answer the fundamental question of who or what I am, and what is the purpose of my life. Like many of my peers in university, at the beginning of the hippie era, I began to explore the magical mysteries of mind-altering drugs, and after graduation, I took this exploration further for another year. This eventually led me to meditation and devoting myself to the practice as a Buddhist monk for eleven years.

Meditation

The word meditation has been used in different contexts to refer to different experiences. The Biblical use refers to a form of prayer in which one reflects on specific thoughts, such as a Bible verse or parable, to reveal their meaning and deepen one's connection with God. The word meditation can even be used to refer to reflection or contemplation on any thought or thought process. When I use the word, I am referring to an ancient technique that for the most part, has been passed on to us from the eastern traditions of Buddhism, Hinduism, Jainism, and Sikhism, and which is the fundamental essence of yoga, the yoking or joining of body, breath, and mind. It is distinct from contemplation or reflection in that thinking is not encouraged. In fact, the primary intention is to let go of thoughts. It is also distinct from the more commonly understood concept of prayer as a conversation with God. However, if prayer is distilled to its essence in which one transcends the duality of considering God as a separate entity or person, then prayer becomes a communion with our divine essence and, as such, has a lot in common with meditation.

The Sanskrit word for meditation is *dhyana*. The Chinese Buddhists translated it as *chan*, the Japanese Buddhists as *zen,* and the Tibetan Buddhists as *gom*. *Dhyana* can be translated as mind vehicle. Meditation uses the mind to go beyond the mind. It is important to understand that this does not mean that meditation requires us to empty the mind of all thoughts. Just as our eyes are meant to see, our ears are meant to hear, our nose is meant to smell and breathe, our tongue is meant to taste, and our body is meant to feel and move, our mind is meant to think. When we meditate, we are not trying to get rid of thoughts or annihilate our minds. So, what do I mean when I say meditation uses the mind to go beyond the mind? Let's examine the process.

Reigning in the Mind

When I sit down to meditate, my primary task is to reign in my mind. One could compare the mind to a wild horse. If I want to tame the horse to ride it and be the master of its movements, the first step is to make friends with it. I need to consciously connect with its mind and body with my mind and body. My whisper to my inner horse is through my breath. The breath is the bridge that allows my mind to connect with my body. The mind side of the bridge is my capacity to control or manipulate the breath with my mind. The body side of the bridge is my body breathing without my mind's intervention. In other words, we can breathe consciously or unconsciously. The thinking mind is, relatively speaking, conscious, whereas the body is unconscious. The intelligence required for the body to harmoniously manage trillions of complex cell interactions is evidence that there is a mind in our body, but this is all going on without the thinking mind's participation. Bridging the gap between the conscious mind and the unconscious body-mind is crucial for inner harmony and wholeness. Tuning into our breath allows us to do that. It is the first step to taming the wild horse.

Finding Your Seat

The body needs to be still and stable to tune in to breath. Meditation is associated with the cross-legged sitting posture of the Buddha, referred to as the lotus pose, because this posture is the ideal position to use as a stable and sustainable foundation for the focus required in meditation. However, not everyone has the hip, knee, and ankle flexibility to sit in this pose comfortably, and it is not essential to sit this way to practice breathwork or pranayama and meditate. The important thing is to sit upright (not leaning back on a chair or wall or crumpled forward). There are various ways to sit cross-legged or kneeling on the floor, usually with a cushion or two for support, and one can even sit in a chair.

Sitting in "cobbler" pose, draw the heels of your feet close to your groins and join the soles of your feet together. If your hips are tight and your knees are now higher than the upper rims of your pelvis, place a firm cushion or folded blanket under your sit bones to elevate the rear of your pelvis. You can see the position of the sit bones over the edge of the cushion in the photo of the kneeling position. This will correct the tendency for your body to fall back behind your center of gravity and help your pelvic "bowl" to tilt forward. This anterior tilt allows the lumbar spine to shift more easily into its natural forward curve, providing the proper angle to support the vertical alignment of the rest of the spinal column.

The pictures that follow show various alternatives.

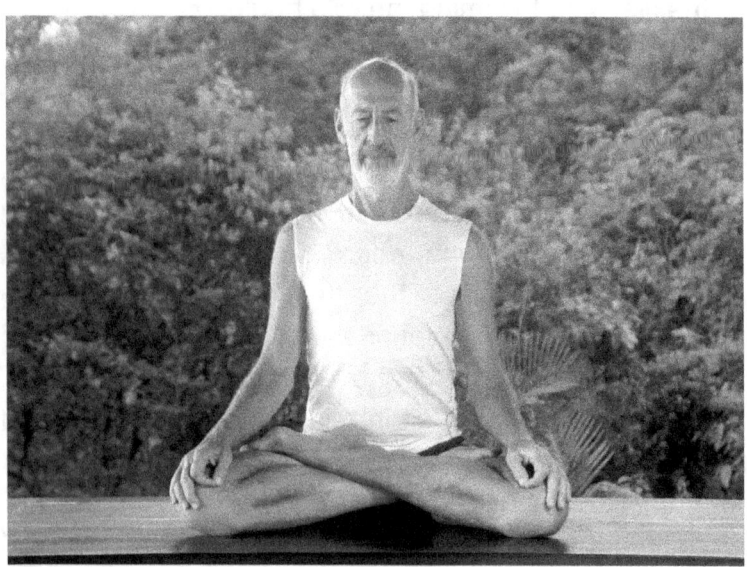

Full Lotus

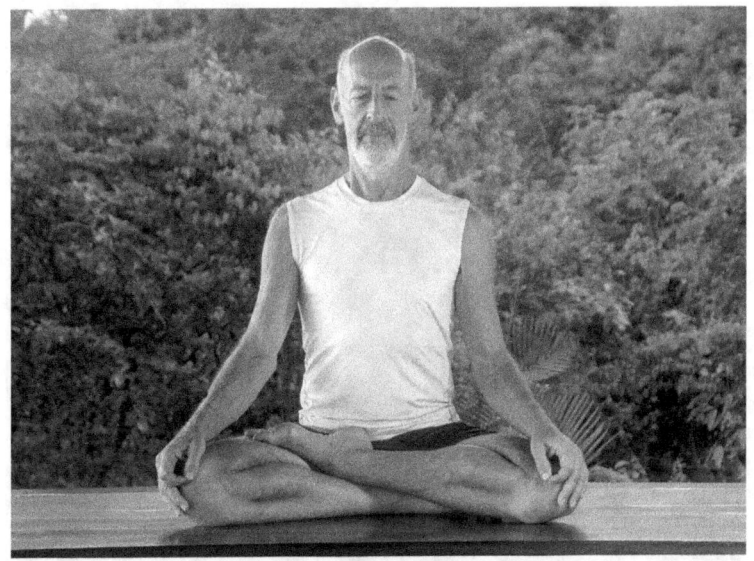

Half Lotus

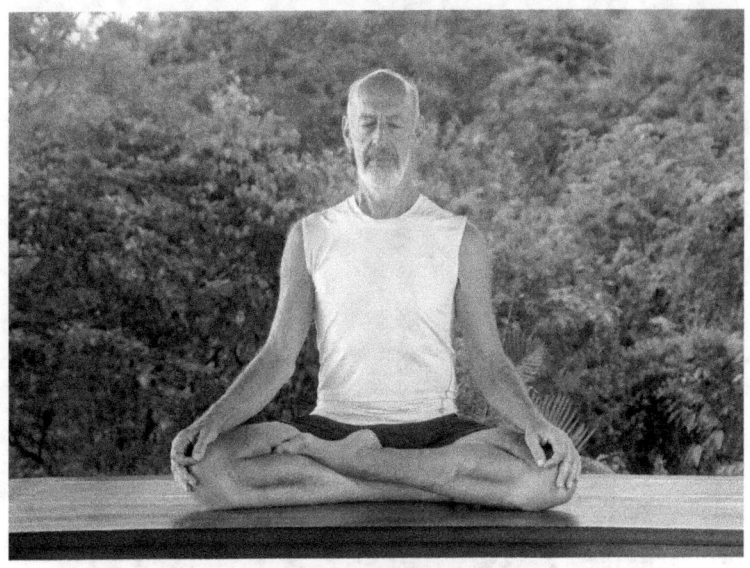

Quarter Lotus

For a more thorough description of achieving this, you can check out my article, *Finding Your Seat,* found on my website: http://voicedialoguemontreal.com/finding-your-seat/.

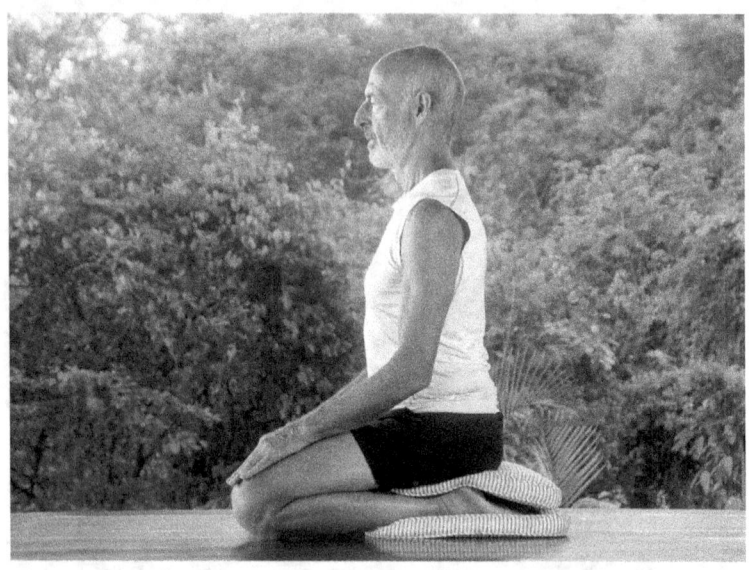
Kneeling Position

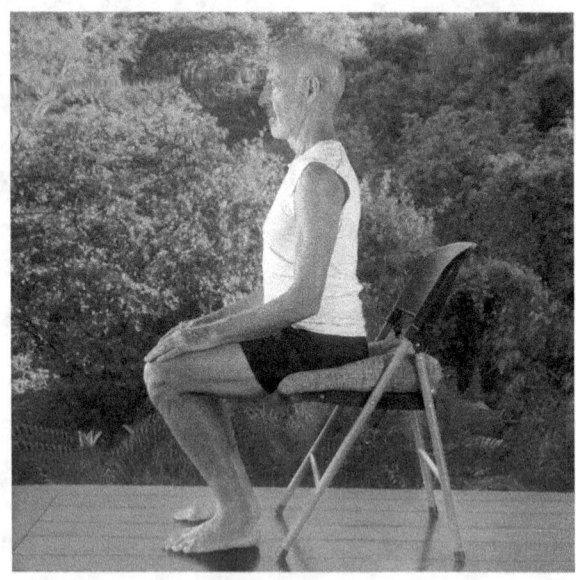
Chair Position

You will notice in the two profile shots that my pelvis is slightly higher than my knees. This allows the pelvis to tilt forward to the ideal position for the spine to find its natural lumbar curve such that the upper body weight is directly over the sit bones in line with gravity. This requires minimum effort to sustain an upright posture that is comfortable and allows freedom of movement of the abdominal diaphragm and no compression of any parts of the spine. This maximizes breath flow and the circulation of chi or vital energy. For most of us, this requires using firm cushions or blocks to elevate the pelvis. When sitting in a chair, make sure to sit close to the edge, away from the back of the chair, and bring the feet as close to you as possible without lifting the heels off the floor to achieve a similar result. For the cross-legged positions, the knees should be firmly grounded; otherwise, the kneeling or chair positions should be used. The idea is to find the most stable and sustainable position to support the steadiness of body and mind.

Calming and Connecting

Begin by simply observing your breath as you breathe in and out through your nose. Don't try to breathe any particular way; just feel how your body responds to your breath's movement. Notice which parts of your body are involved in this movement. Notice the rhythm of your breath without judgment or trying to change it. Your breath may be very shallow or deep and full. It may be quick, choppy, smooth, slow, rhythmic, labored, or easy. How you breathe at any given moment reflects your mental and emotional state. Simply giving attention to your breath by following its course in and out with a curious beginner's mind will gradually temper its expression towards ease as energy enjoys the path of least resistance.

Once you have settled into your breath in this way, count how long it takes for you to breathe in and out without trying to modify your natural breath. You can mentally count "AUM 1, AUM 2, etc." to ensure a regular pace. After 5 to 10 breaths, you will notice a pattern. For example, 4 counts for the breath in and 3 counts for the breath out, or 3 counts for the breath in and 4 counts for the breath out. There is no right or wrong here. Just observe. Now extend your exhalations to twice as long as your inhalations. So, if you are breathing in to the count of 4, breathe out to the count of 8. Extending the exhalation in this way will require some effort. Instead of letting the air fall out, contract the belly inward to push residual air out of your lungs, like squeezing a sponge to expel all the water. In the same way that no effort is required when you release the squeeze on the sponge to fill up with air and resume its expanded state, release the contraction to allow the air coming in to fill the space you have created. Continue breathing like this for about 5 minutes.

Now allow your breath to subside to your new natural breathing rhythm and notice what you feel. Extending the exhalations, as you have just done, calms the nervous system, so you will likely feel quite peaceful and calm. If you wish, you can continue to sit and observe your breath. Thoughts tend to take our attention away from our breath and agitate the breath or cause us to disconnect into a dreamy and sleepy state, so you can add a mental focus and take this into meditation. Simply continue to observe your breath's flow and notice thoughts as they arise without allowing them to take over. You can simply let each thought go with each exhalation. Simply following the breath is your fundamental tool for meditation.

My thoughts are like satellites and space particles spinning around Mother Earth, each drawing my attention to their orbital paths. Like a yoyo in a "round the world" move, they are each held in their orbit by a kind of gravitational string of attraction, sharing a common hub at the center of me, the experiencer. This energetic pattern appears to repeat itself in everything inside and around me, down to the tiniest atom with its electrons spinning around its nucleus. Reigning in my mind back to its nucleus at the center of my being is the aspect of meditation we call concentration— bringing our focus back to the center.

We are using the power of our mind to re-mind itself of who it is and who we are at home base. We are not trying to jump off the merry-go-round but rather find our way back to its core—the generator and experiencer of the thoughts.

One could say that the point of concentration in meditation is to shift our focus from being carried away by the peripheral projections of the mind and get back into the driver's seat at the source of it all. Good and bad things and everything in between will always happen, but when we are rooted in our source at the center of it all, we will no longer be overwhelmed by our circumstances.

Breathwork

Arguably breathwork deserves to be at the forefront of any discussion about the essentials for the wholeness of body and mind. We can debate what or how much we need to eat, sleep, exercise, practice meditation, or any other discipline, but no one will dispute the fundamental importance of breathing. I have waited until now to introduce this subject because I trust that I don't need to remind anyone to breathe while they hear about other healthy habits to practice for a fulfilling life, as our autonomic nervous system takes care of this and other essential functions. However, like eating, exercise, and other practices, how we breathe and how much we breathe significantly impacts the quality of our life and how long we live.

Breath is distinct from other functions in the body in that it can function on its own, but we can also consciously manipulate it. As such, it acts as a bridge between our relatively unconscious body that operates without our telling our heart to pump blood or our digestive system to digest food or our relatively conscious mind that thinks (ideally) before speaking or acting. The fact that breath lies at the critical juncture between mind and body justifies introducing breathwork in the context of self-knowledge. Mastery of the breath is an art that requires our full attention and considerable practice, but the benefits for our body, mind, and spirit are well worth it. It is also appropriate to introduce it after introducing the practice of meditation, as it facilitates and empowers one's capacity to meditate.

Pranayama

As mentioned earlier, *prana* is the Sanskrit word for life force, called *chi* in the Chinese martial arts or *ki* in the Japanese martial arts. *Ayama* means expansion. So, pranayama literally expands your life force. Pranayama is an integral part of yoga practice and is the fourth of the eight limbs (*ashtanga*) of yoga. The eight limbs or branches of yoga describe the progression of a complete yoga practice. The first two limbs are the *yamas*, and the *niyamas*, the personal observances to live well. Briefly, the *yamas* describe how to behave outwardly toward the world, and the *yamas* how to behave inwardly towards yourself. The third limb is the practice of *asana*, literally translated as seat, which refers to the physical performance of postures, which in modern times is commonly referred to as yoga, or Hatha yoga, from which all the "yoga" schools have sourced their systems.

The *asanas* bring awareness to your body. With this foundation, one is prepared for the fourth limb *pranayama,* which brings awareness to your breath. As breath connects the body with the mind, this awareness prepares us for the fifth limb of *pratyahara*, which refers to the withdrawal of our senses, or to put it another way, shifting our focus from the objects of our senses to their source within. The senses tend to disperse our attention outwardly and foster the illusion that happiness or contentment is to be found outside oneself. The practice of *pratyahara* trains the mind to discover or rediscover the source of contentment where the senses originate within. Once the mind is brought back into focus, we are ready to practice the sixth limb of *dharana*, or concentration. When this one-pointed concentration is sustained, we practice *dhyana* (chan in Chinese, zen in Japanese) or meditation, which can be described as letting go of all distractions to be fully present. The practice and integration of all the above eventually lead us to be established in complete surrender of all duality, the illusion of self and other, to realize our Oneness, the eighth and final limb of yoga called *samadhi*.

Though these limbs are described as successive stages, built on each other, they can and will be experienced in any order and various degrees and influence and enhance each other accordingly.

Many breathing techniques qualify as pranayama both within the classical yoga tradition and similar traditions such as Chi Gung, Taoist yoga, and even in contemporary approaches, including sports or performing arts, each with their particular benefits. I shall share a simple and accessible sequence that is quite comprehensive in its benefits. It concludes with a deep breathing technique that empowers the practitioner to perform such feats as extended breath retention and to tolerate extreme conditions such as ice-cold temperatures with no warm clothing, popularized by Wim Hoff, the "Ice Man." I recommend this sequence be done only after regular practice of the preceding exercises. I include it here not so much for practicing extreme feats but more fundamentally because it is perhaps the most powerful thing, we can do to ensure optimal body and mind function and even help heal emotional disease. Though it can be practiced almost any time, I practice this sequence every day in the half-hour preceding my morning meditation because, as I mentioned earlier, it facilitates and energizes one's meditation practice.

Pranayama Exercises

First, these exercises should be practiced on an empty or half-full stomach. If you must eat prior to practicing pranayama, eat lightly.

Wear comfortable clothing that is not tight around the waist and does not hamper the movement of the diaphragm.

It is important to sit in a comfortable posture with a straight back. Assume the same posture you use for meditation.

All of us have a habitual breathing pattern reflecting and affecting our attitude. Some are belly breathers, some tend to hold their belly in and breathe only in the chest, some emphasize inhalations, some emphasize exhalations, some have a short and shallow breathing pattern, and some take long slow breaths. Some have a hurried breath, and some hold or hesitate when they breathe, and, of course, our breath fluctuates with our moods or reaction to circumstances. Yogic breath is a full breath, including the participation of the belly, the lower ribcage, and the upper chest and back ribs. In the beginning, preparing our breathing mechanism for full breaths is helpful by practicing the three-part breath.

Three-Part Breath

Use a few cushions to create a small hill. Lie down on the cushions and make sure that the resulting stretch of the back is very comfortable. No tension should be felt whatsoever. Watch your breath and let it follow its natural course and rhythm, then begin to count your in-breaths and try to slow down your out-breaths until they become twice as long as the in-breaths. Breathe through the nose. First, breathe in from the abdomen; then fill up the lower rib cage, followed by the upper rib cage underneath the collar bone. Breathing out is done in the same order starting from the diaphragm. Be aware of your back. Allow it to widen with the breath in.

This exercise is a great help in facilitating proper breathing from the diaphragm. It increases lung capacity.

Sequence of Eight Pranayamas

Resume an upright sitting posture.

1. **Nadi Shodona** (1:4:2 alternate nostril breathing)
   This precedes the eight other breathing exercises.

   - Breathe in through the right nostril, closing the left nostril with the middle finger of the right hand.

Mentally count AUM 1, AUM 2, etc., to know how long it takes to complete your inhalation.

- Close the right nostril with the thumb of the right hand. Hold the air in up to four times as long as it took for you to breathe in, counting at the same pace as you counted to breathe in.

- Remove the middle finger and breathe out through the left nostril, extending the exhalation twice as long as it took for you to breathe in.

- Breathe in through the left nostril, counting as before, then close the left nostril and hold the air in, again four times as long as it took to breathe in.

- Breathe out through the right nostril and start again at step 1

- Repeat this alternate nostril breath for 10 to 20 breaths

- Complete the sequence by breathing in through the right nostril and breathing out through the left nostril.

This exercise helps to balance the left and right channels, so you can take more time if you need to equalize the flow of breath and energy through the two nostrils. The left channel facilitates the flow of feminine energy of receptivity or being, and the right activates the masculine energy of doing.

Benefits:

- Infuses the body with oxygen
- Clears and releases toxins
- Reduces stress and anxiety
- Calms and rejuvenates the nervous system
- Helps to balance hormones
- Supports clear and balanced respiratory channels
- Helps to alleviate respiratory allergies that cause hay fever, sneezing, or wheezing
- The attention you give to the different actions also helps to prepare you to concentrate during meditation

2. **Ütjè Kumbhack** (one cycle)
- Breathe in through both nostrils.
- Close both nostrils and hold the air four times as long.
- Breathe out through the left nostril twice as long.

Benefits:

- Cures diseases caused by phlegm

3. **Shîtkâr Kumbhack** (one cycle)
- Breathe in through both nostrils.
- Hold the air in four times as long.
- Breathe out, whistling twice as long.

Benefits:
- Alleviates hunger and thirst

4. **Shîtalî Kumbhack** (one cycle)

A. Breathe in through the mouth with the tongue sticking out.
- Hold your breath four times as long.
- Breathe out through both nostrils twice as long.

B. Fold your tongue in half to resemble a beak and breathe in.
- Hold your breath four times as long.
- Breathe out through both nostrils twice as long.

Benefits:
- Cures diseases caused by spleen

5. **Bhastrika Kumbhack** (bellows breath)

This pranayama is quite powerful. Do not repeat more than twice in a row and no more than four times, six hours apart.

- Breathe in through both nostrils.

- Breathe out through both nostrils, pulling the abdomen in, emphasize the breath out.

- Keep breathing in this manner, accelerating the rhythm of the breath gradually. You can work your way up to 108x.

- Breathe in through the right nostril, filling the entire breathing cavity.

- Hold the air inside as long as you are comfortable to hold without forcing.

- With eyes closed, place the attention on a point about 12 inches in front of the middle of the forehead.

- Breathe out through the left nostril.

6. **Bhrâmarî Kumbhack** (bee breath)

- Breathe in through both nostrils.

- Hold four times as long.

- Breathe out, humming twice as long.

7. **Ujjayi Pranayama** (cobra breath)

- First, to engage the three locks or *bandhas*, extend your exhalation through the nose to squeeze all the air out and contract the belly deep into the spine. Holding the air out, engage the root lock (*mula bandha*) by contracting the perineum (the muscle between the vagina or testicles and the anus) inward and upward, as if you are holding in an urgent need to pee.

- Hold this lock and add the contraction of the abdominal diaphragm just below the rib cage (*uddiyana bandha*) by sucking the belly upward into the rib cage.

- Finally, tuck in the chin to engage the throat lock (*jalandhara bandha*). All three locks should be performed while keeping the spine upright.

- Keeping all three locks engaged, take a deep breath in through the nose. As your abdomen is not releasing to create space for the lungs to descend into as they inflate, the ribcage is forced to expand both in the front and back, creating an effect similar to a cobra flaring out its upper body as it assumes its erect posture. This is part of why the Sanskrit name for this pranayama is *ujjayi*, which can be translated as victorious inner stretching.

- As soon as you come to the top of the breath, exhale without hesitating, still holding all three locks, and continue breathing in and out through the nose without pausing at the end of the in-breath or out-breath. There will be a tendency to relax the contractions, especially the lower two, as the body attempts to find space to breathe into or during the transition into exhaling because of the habit of relaxing on the out-breath to resist that tendency. This requires constant effort and concentration. Because of the constriction in the throat, each breath in and out should sound like the ocean or the sound of a conch shell held close to your ear.

- Repeat 5 or 6 times.

Ujjayi breathing quiets the brain, increases oxygenation, and slows the flow of breathing. It regulates the body's internal heat, helps control blood pressure, and releases tension. It also strengthens the digestive and nervous systems.

8. **Kevalya Kumbhack** (breath of non-attachment)
- Allow your breath to subside to its natural flow in and out through the nose. Observe its flow and notice if you are emphasizing either your in-breath or out-breath and if there is any pause in your breathing cycle.

- See if you can eliminate the pause at the top of the inhalation or the bottom of the exhalation. In other words, visualize your breath as an infinite loop rather than a square box with corners, a top, a bottom, and sides. The in-breath makes a seamless transition into the out-breath, and the out-breath makes a seamless transition into the in-breath.

- Continuing to breathe in this way will result in an increasingly subtle breath such that, at some point, it may be difficult to sense if you are breathing in or out, and you may even reach a state of equanimity in which it seems that you are not even breathing at all. This is not holding the breath but more like a natural suspension of the breath. Prana is still circulating and being absorbed, i.e., there is still an energetic flow, but the physical movement of the breathing mechanism becomes virtually imperceptible.

- If you have stopped breathing and need to reinitiate movement to get more oxygen, do so gently so as not to create agitation and to maintain the ease of this exercise.

- Breathe as if you were breathing through the cheeks and the eyes.

9. **20-20-20 Fractionalized In-Breath**

- Breathe into your belly through both nostrils and hold for 20 seconds. Engage the root lock (*mula bandha*).

- Inhale again, this time focusing the breath in the chest area to inflate the ribcage and hold another 20 seconds, adding the contraction of your abdominal diaphragm (*uddiyana bandha*) to the root lock.

- Inhale one more time, this time visualizing the breath filling your cranium, and hold another 20 seconds, adding the throat lock (*jaladhara bandha*) by tucking in the chin.

- Breathe out and relax, breathing in and out freely.

This sequence can be practiced first thing in the morning to prepare your body-mind for the day or meditation. It is also an excellent warm-up session for the dynamic deep breathing practice described in the following section.

Controlled Hyperventilation Technique

The following exercise is a powerful breathing technique that creates a hyperventilation effect that decreases the carbon dioxide level and raises the PH in your blood. It is like the breathing techniques free divers use to expand their capacity to suspend their breath under water and adapt to the stress of atmospheric pressure changes. Wim Hoff has developed this method and made it popular by demonstrating extreme feats of withstanding ice-cold temperatures and setting several record-breaking athletic endeavors, such as swimming under ice caps, climbing Mount Everest and Kilimanjaro with just a bathing suit and shoes, running barefoot half-marathons on snow, and running a marathon in the desert without water.

Though Wim Hoff appears to be eccentric and intense in his character, much scientific research has substantiated his claims and those of practitioners of his method that seem to combine pranayama techniques with the Tibetan *tummo* meditation practiced by advanced yogis. In addition to the benefits of pranayama previously described, this dynamic breathing exercise induces a short stress response that stimulates the body's capacity to heal diseases due to a compromised immune system and gives it more resilience to deal with everyday stress, both physically and mentally. There are more specific claims about its effect on physical and mental health, many of which are substantiated by scientific researchers, that I will leave you to research online or elsewhere and make your own conclusions. Some of this information has influenced me but what has made me a believer and a daily practitioner is my personal experience.

So, what happens to the body during Wim Hof breathing?

When we breathe in, we take up oxygen and release carbon dioxide from our blood. Our blood is usually fully saturated with oxygen (about 99% saturation) and deep breathing does not raise that saturation. Deep breathing does, however, release a lot of carbon dioxide. This, in turn, lowers the "urge to breathe."

The brain stem, specifically the pons and medulla oblongata, is sensitive to carbon dioxide. Having too much carbon dioxide in the blood will trigger your brain stem to breathe. By removing carbon dioxide from the blood through deep breathing, this impulse to breathe from the brain stem is lowered. In short, the lower the level of carbon dioxide, the longer you can hold your breath. The impulse is just not triggered yet.

Furthermore, by systematically and deeply breathing in and out, the pH value in the blood increases (making the blood more alkaline), whereas the acidity lessens. Normally, on average, the pH value is 7.4. By exerting the breathing techniques, this becomes significantly higher and can even go up to 7.75. As a result, three important physiological changes happen: You can experience lightheadedness as the arteries and veins to the brain and body close slightly in reaction to the alkalizing blood. You can experience a tingling sensation in the limbs and muscles due to the lowering of the available calcium ions in the blood. Removing free calcium ions increases muscle excitability. The red blood cells carrying oxygen have a difficult time releasing their payload of oxygen. Why? Because acidity normally triggers the release. If the blood is too alkaline, the oxygen bound to the red blood cell does not release. This makes the cells and tissues unable to receive oxygen even though blood oxygen saturation is at 100%. The oxygen is simply "stuck" to the red blood cell. This is also known as "Hypoxia," defined as a deficiency in the amount of oxygen reaching the tissues.

This might sound scary, but this mild hypoxic state caused by the controlled deep breathing is soon back to normal again. At the final deep breath, breathing out and holding the breath will allow the blood to re-establish acidity and allow red blood cells to begin releasing their oxygen. While holding the breath, no new oxygen comes back into the blood. As a result, oxygen saturation in the blood lowers as the body uses it up. Remember, there is also less carbon dioxide, which makes breath-holding easier as well!

The body is now experiencing a short-term form of hypoxia, a form of stress at the cellular level. Cells are not getting normal oxygen levels, and their metabolism begins to shift. This stress will signal the body to react and strengthen. The body's sympathetic responses are activated, and the pathways necessary to deliver that oxygen to cells are strengthened. These pathways could include several different systems, such as increasing red blood cells, increasing lung capacity, improving circulation, and improving metabolic efficiency over the long term.

This short-term period of hypoxia is a positive stressor. It signals the body to react and strengthen and to better deal with stress in the long term. How does this work?

Let's look at Radboud's endotoxin study (2014), which measured trained participants performing the breathing technique. Their blood first alkalized through the breathing, then acidified during the breath hold, releasing oxygen to the tissue and lowering blood oxygen saturation. The breathing technique was performed for multiple rounds, lowering blood oxygen saturation at every round!

Another interesting physiological effect of the breathing method is the increased adrenaline level in the blood. The Radboud study recorded such large amounts of adrenaline in its participants that it is speculated that the breathing method influenced the adrenal medulla, located in the adrenal gland. This is one of the most abundant sources of adrenaline in the body and, given the elevated levels the study recorded in the participants, it would make sense that the breathing method influenced this important sympathetic response—an influence we didn't think was possible before the Radboud study! [22]

In short, this self-induced hyperventilation technique creates a hypoxic state in the body that acts as a positive stressor to shift the metabolism and stimulate the body's systems to produce an anti-inflammatory response and strengthen the immune system.

What follows are clear step-by-step instructions that describe how I practice it, including some fine-tuning and more attention to detail than you will find in most online sources meant to be introductory. Before attempting to do this exercise, prepare your body-mind by practicing the preceding pranayama exercises for at least a few weeks daily. I also recommend that once you start the Wim Hoff breathing technique, you precede the practice with the eight-part pranayama sequence, which will empower your capacity for more effective breaths and breath retentions and decrease the probability of any negative effects from the hyperventilation.

---

[22] https://www.wimhofmethod.com/breathing-exercises

I have been practicing it daily for about a few years, and I have not experienced any immediate or long-term negative effects. On the contrary, starting my day with this practice supercharges my meditation following the breathwork and has a definite uplifting effect on my body, mind, and spirit. This effect lasts for hours and has a cumulative effect on my well-being when practiced regularly. I have practiced pranayama breathing techniques regularly for most of my life, so I recommend starting with a qualified instructor who can guide and observe you to give you feedback on how you are performing the actions.

IMPORTANT: *Do not practice the following hyperventilation and breath retention exercises while driving a vehicle or doing any activity where fainting would be dangerous. Do not practice retention under water unless you are accompanied by a qualified practitioner or instructor monitoring you closely.*

Also, if you have high blood pressure, check with your cardiologist whether it is safe to practice these exercises. If your blood pressure has been normalized with medication, there should be no problem. In fact, you may find that your pressure will lower with regular practice.

Here we go!

First, as with the other breathing exercises described earlier, this practice should be practiced on an empty stomach and in a stable and comfortable sitting posture. The following exercises can be practiced lying down on your back, which has some advantages to help the body release tensions by surrendering all the muscles to gravity when you have suspended the breathing for the retentions. However, I recommend first doing them sitting in a vertical position because it makes it easier to perform the spinal undulation, which facilitates the continuity of breath and energy flow called kundalini by the yogis up and down the channels between the seven chakras from the root chakra (pelvic floor) to the crown chakra (top of the head). Kundalini refers to the serpent-like energy that resides at the bottom of the spine like a coiled-up snake. When it is awakened, it spirals upwards and can be felt as an inner bliss that starts in the spine and circulates through your body. Deep breathing will activate it, especially when it is assisted by an undulating movement between the pelvis and head. Therefore, I combine this wave-like motion while doing the hyperventilation. As you are not in front of me for me to demonstrate, I will describe the movement below.

To maximize the easy flow of breath, we breathe through the mouth, in and out, during hyperventilation. First, take a deep breath in, arching upwards with your chest, arms out a little and relaxed and head dropping back a little to create a "C" shape. Then as you exhale, reverse the "C" so that you are bending forward into your own body, with your chest and head dropping towards your legs and shoulders rounding slightly as the passive arms follow. Here, you are creating space in the chest for the lungs to receive the maximum amount of air in the inhalation. The shoulders should not be pulled back as this will contract the upper back muscles and restrict the expansion of the back of the rib cage. On the exhalation, the forward collapsing motion helps to expel the air like compressing a bellows pump.

While these two "C" shapes facilitate the inflow and outflow of the breath, there is a better option. Imagine the two opposite "C" formations morphing into "S" shapes intersecting at your diaphragm and joining to form figure 8. The shape of figure 8 is the symbol of infinity for a good reason. It is continuous without interruption. When your breath flows through this pathway, it will be continuous with no interruption or pause between the in-breath and the out-breath and vice versa. This is what we are looking for maximum efficacy of hyperventilation.

If you are not used to that movement, which is an undulation from the pelvis to your head, this might help: Initiate the arching forward from the pelvic area by tipping your pelvis forward as you breathe in. Allowing your upper body to relax and follow will send your chest forward, and your head will flop backward. Then when you exhale, once again, initiate the movement from the pelvis, this time tipping the pelvis in the opposite direction by tucking in the tailbone. This will push the lower back from the arched position to round backward, and the upper body should follow with the chest dropping downward to your legs and the head dropping forward toward your chest. Continue this wave-like movement back and forth in rhythm with your breath, arching forward as you inhale and curling backward as you exhale.

I usually precede the hyperventilation with the eight pranayamas because, apart from having their own benefits, they prepare your body-mind for this powerful technique. The first four increase breath flow and lung capacity, then the bellows, or fire breaths, get your body moving into the undulations and your breath according to the motion. It also fans the flame of the inner fire to melt the crystallizations of habitual holding patterns and to create more space in your core. Then the extended hum of the bee breath (*bhramari*) vibrates the core right down to the pelvic floor to establish your root lock for the succeeding ujaayii breaths, and the ujaayi breaths tone the core and lengthen the body to provide support for efficient hyperventilation. Finally, the 20-20-20 inhalation breath-hold creates the space to maximize your capacity for quick and full breath intakes in the hyperventilation sequence.

However, if you don't have the time to do the preliminary pranayamas, at least start with the 20-20-20-inhalation breath-hold before each hyperventilation sequence. Then immediately following the exhalation, begin breathing in and out through your mouth to maximize the inflow and outflow of breath. Do not allow yourself to pause at the top of your in-breath or the bottom of your out-breath. This is challenging at first as we don't breathe like this naturally unless we run uphill, do a circuit of intense exercises, or recover from a sprint. This is similar in terms of the rhythm bit without the panting. Here we are not desperately gasping for oxygen; we are simply eliminating the pauses between breaths. However, not taking the time to absorb the breath in or linger passively after exhaling can feel like we are being pushed, creating anxiety and tension. This can limit our capacity to take in more oxygen and expel more carbon dioxide, which is the purpose of hyperventilation.

To avoid this tendency, visualize your breath as a continuous stream flowing in coordination with the undulating movement of your torso described earlier. Instead of a distinct rise and fall of in-breath and out-breath, it is more like circular breathing where the in-breath gently transitions into the out-breath and the out-breath into the in-breath. Properly done, the continuous movement describes a figure 8 which is appropriately the symbol for infinity. It should feel like a graceful dance; the smoother it gets, the quieter it gets. Though it is quite forceful and stimulating to sustain this rhythm through the cycle of breaths, the momentum of the undulations and movement of the breath minimizes the physical effort. The effort is primarily in the attention you give to sustain the subtle flow rather than fall into a less conscious breathing pattern. At first, this may feel awkward, but with regular practice, you will be able to refine the movement and enjoy smoother and fuller breathing, which will enhance your capacity to hold your breath as well.

Keep your breath moving in this way for 30 breaths. Then, without forcing all the air out, close your mouth after the last exhalation and refrain from breathing in. Suspend your breathing for as long as you can. Relax every muscle in your body, including your face, jaw, and tongue. You may feel some contractions in your diaphragm or chest. Some of that is due to fear, anxiety or panic. This can occur not long after the beginning of the breath hold or when you start thinking about terminating the breath hold. You can just observe the contraction and let it go. You will likely be surprised that sooner or later, you feel very calm and experience no urge to breathe, and the contraction doesn't recur for a considerable length of time as you have just decreased the level of carbon dioxide in your blood, which inhibits this survival reflex. However, later, towards the end of your capacity to hold, there can be a physiological reflex that causes some spasms in the diaphragm. If you allow those contractions to happen and continue to hold your breath a little longer, it feels like you get a second breath, and can hold a little longer. During a freediving course in Thailand, my instructor explained why this occurs. I do not recall the physiological description, but it has something to do with an endocrine reaction that gives a message to the body's systems to relax their functions to favor available oxygen to go primarily to the brain. Yes, the body has its hierarchy!

When you reach the end of your holding capacity, take a deep breath in, exhale, then take another breath in and hold for 20-60 seconds, allowing your body to drink in the nourishing oxygen. Then exhale and allow your breath to flow in and out naturally. If you want to do another cycle of 30 hyperventilations and breath retention, warm up first with another 20-20-20 fractionalized inhalation. You can also eventually increase the number of hyperventilations to 60 for the second cycle and 90 for the third cycle. However, I suggest you wait until you have experienced the effect of this practice for a few days before adding more repetitions. When you do, start by adding a cycle or two of 30 breaths before increasing to 60 and 90. You will find that you can hold your breath longer after the second cycle, especially if you increase the number of hyperventilations. I can hold for 30 seconds longer after the second cycle and a minute longer after the third.

These exercises will also prepare your body for other activities that create positive stress on your body's systems, such as bathing in ice-cold water or performing an athletic feat. The hypothermic effect of bathing in ice-cold water is a positive stressor that will also strengthen your immune system and amp up your metabolism. You can start with just taking cold showers and gradually experimenting with colder temperatures. Again, use your common sense not to attempt potentially dangerous activities, especially not without qualified supervision. For most of us, the purpose of these exercises is not to see if we can break the Guinness Book of World Records for breath-holding or doing extreme sports. They are offered here as part of my sharing with you what I do to live a more fulfilling life. I do these daily, and without a doubt, they inspire my body, mind, and spirit. They are also one of the best things you can do to fortify your physical health, decrease or eliminate depression, energize your creative projects, and tap into your blissful and peaceful essence. When my day doesn't turn out quite the way I or some part of me would have liked, if it includes a good breathing and meditation session, I'm good!

7
Inner Work

The vision of oneness allows no real separation between our inner and outer experience. By outer experience I am referring to what we consciously perceive during our waking hours occurring in our body-mind, whether perceived as tangible events or experiences with independent existence or as mental-emotional thoughts and memories within our psyche of which we have conscious awareness. Inner experience refers to the corresponding realm of experience that lies beneath the surface of our conscious mind, or what a dear friend of mine called the surface-level thinking mind. Carl Jung called this inner realm the unconscious. While we cannot hope to perceive and control everything that happened to us, is happening to us, or will happen to us, if we are to live an integrated and fulfilling life, we cannot limit our awareness to the so-called outer reality. Our experience of outer reality is intimately connected with our inner reality. The fact that we are unaware of the unconscious realm of experience does not make it any less real or significant. The mind can be compared to the ocean. The surface of the ocean is vast. Think of this as the surface-level thinking mind that operates during the waking state. At the surface, we may see waves, people surfing or swimming between them, pelicans diving into them to snatch fish swimming close to the surface, boats moving over the surface, and plenty of things floating on the surface. However, miles beneath the surface lies a far vaster space full of life that exists whether we are aware of it or not. Think of this as the subconscious or unconscious mind. We have access to this realm when we dream, and when information or energies penetrate the filters of the ego-mind through various practices we can perform in the waking state or in states that transcend the waking state. However, before we examine how we can dive beneath the surface level thinking mind, we can ask ourselves: Why should we bother? For many of us, our dream life has little or no relevance or use in our daily lives in the waking state. For many, psychotherapy that digs beneath our surface experience is "for crazy people, not me." When we are relatively comfortable identifying with our "normal" reality, the various techniques or practices that alter our state of body and mind to transcend "normal" reality can threaten our habitual and familiar realm of experience.

Yes, we should bother because, as the ocean metaphor suggests, what lies beneath the surface profoundly affects what occurs at the surface. Ironically, avoiding or ignoring our inner world to maintain a semblance of control in our lives has exactly the opposite effect. We can only hope to control or at least manage what we are conscious of. What lies below the radar of our conscious mind is out of our control. It also has control over us without our being aware of it. What we don't own owns us. When the filters of our conscious ego-mind do not allow these energies to express themselves, they will sneak into our lives in surreptitious ways. This will be described more thoroughly in this chapter. I am not suggesting that we should constantly relive or remember everything we have experienced. Several years ago, I read an interesting article that offered an alternate perspective in response to the marketing of supplements or devices claiming improved memory in their list of benefits. The writer said that he was not sure he would want to remember everything that he had experienced in his life. The fact that our memory is selective has its benefits. We do not need or want to relive unpleasant or painful experiences. However, as shall be described in the theory of subpersonalities in the following section, we, or more particularly the ego-mind we call "me," is itself a product of the impressions engraved in our memory bank, so it does not always process these experiences or our memories of them in ways that serve us.

Voice Dialogue and the Theory of Subpersonalities

While we usually conceive of the self as singular, we have several parts that make up who we are. We are a collection of selves. Our personality is a combination of subpersonalities. The theory of subpersonalities that I shall share with you here was developed by Hal and Sidra Stone, my teachers and mentors in the Voice Dialogue method, which they developed in the 1980s and which has profoundly influenced my life and thousands of others in the years that followed.

The psychology of selves is as old as Freud's concepts of id, ego, and superego and is addressed in several psycho-therapeutic methods. The Voice Dialogue method is a relatively new technique for physically and energetically separating the selves from the ego. Developed by the late and his wife in the 1980's, it is a blend of several different therapeutic systems: Gestalt, Jungian, Psychosynthesis, Transactional Analysis, and psychodrama.

Where do personalities come from? The kind of parents we have and the circumstances we are born into play an important role in forming the personalities we develop in our efforts to cope with our emergence into this world. However, we know from nature versus nurture research that we are born with some personality characteristics. This was confirmed for me when I witnessed my daughter's birth. Her eyes were wide open as if to say: "The world is my apple!" This characteristic has certainly proved evident in how she has manifested herself in this life. It is reasonable to surmise that the inherent tendencies particular to each individual, whether inherited genetically or as part of a karmic process that transcends their current incarnation, influence different individuals born into very similar circumstances to make very different choices and consequently develop and display different personality characteristics.

Here is the basic theory of how this process takes place. We are all born vulnerable with little or no knowledge or experience in this life of how to fend for ourselves. Our five senses may be intact, but our capacity to interpret our experience, let alone know what strategies will serve to protect us or get us what we need, has yet to be discovered. For example, a newborn infant feels discomfort in its belly but does not know it is hungry. Then mama offers her breast to feed it some warm and sweet milk, and the discomfort is allayed. That feels good! Discomfort gone. I would like more of that! A desire is born, and with that, the association between comfort and mama. Various behaviors develop in relation to that association. Most babies will cry when they are uncomfortable. As this usually gets the caregiver's attention, the memory of this can reinforce this behavior, so until they learn new ways to express their feelings or needs, the infant does this to get their wants or needs met. For some, this behavior can persist after the infant or even child has learned other ways to express themselves. This can lay the foundation for a pattern of negative attention-getting that can persist even into adult life. One example would be using drama to get what one wants. Another would be complaining rather than just asking for what one wants. An extreme version of this is to threaten to commit suicide and sometimes even follow through with it to various degrees when one is desperately reaching out for help. On the other hand, many of us discover alternate ways designed to get positive attention, such as smiling.

A baby spontaneously smiles when it is experiencing pleasure and receives a positive response from its caregiver or the person in front of them. This association encourages the development of a pleaser persona. *Persona* comes from Greek. *Sona* means sound, and *per* means through. *Per-sona* literally translates as sound-through. In ancient Greek, theatre actors wore masks to portray the roles they were playing. The sounds came through their masks. *Persona* was the word for a mask. The smiling face will eventually develop into such behavior as telling people what you think they want to hear in the hope that they will like you or give you what you want. Conversely, a frowning face or expressing anger will let them know you are not happy with their behavior. Masks will not only express or convey the expression of the character they represent but also act as layers concealing other characters behind the primary or dominant mask or persona. For example, we may be concealing the frowning mask behind the smiling mask so as not to repel the person we are interacting with by revealing the part of ourselves that is displeased. The truth is that we are not just one self. We are many selves, many personas or masks. Masks are not false selves, but they are partial. They are aspects of our whole self, each with their own character and agenda. Some examples of personas or selves are the Controller-Protector, the Inner Critic, the Pusher, the Vulnerable Child, the Playful Child, the Clown, the Judge, the Responsible Father, the Nurturing Mother, the Guru, the Teacher, the Caregiver, the Therapist, and the list goes on. These are names for commonly occurring selves, but we each have a unique collection. We share archetypes like the Savior, the Hero, the Warrior, etc., in our collective psyche. The ancient Greeks seem to have understood this in their honoring a multiplicity of Gods. As long as we are going to personify

God, why would we restrict him or her to one persona? It would make sense that a universal God has many expressions or energetics. What makes us unique is not only which selves make up our ego complex but with which we more or less identified.

Mama does not just offer comfort. She offers a loving connection. Comfort is a more fear-based experience that implies being relieved or sheltered from an uncomfortable state. The fear-based experience will evolve into desire as we seek to obtain and enjoy that experience again. Both fear and desire are rooted in our sense of separation, which is the fundamental ignorance at the root of all suffering. In love's purest expression, there is no sense of separation. Love is the ultimate connection we all seek. What is the purest expression of love? Oneness. No sense of other, absence of fear, absence of need, complete fulfillment. When we are separated at birth from the oneness of being inside our mother, the heroic journey back to the source of oneness begins. Upon emerging from the womb, it is not only our umbilical connection with our mother that is cut. Whereas before, we did not know ourselves as other than our mother's body, we are catapulted into a world of otherness, where we are a separate self among others. We first learn how to recognize ourselves as separate beings and develop skills to ensure the survival of our separate egos. The human paradox is that this engenders the drama of human suffering, yet what keeps us going is the longing to find our way back to the fulfillment of our original wholeness, the One that knows no other.

In the early days of my career as a massage therapist and bodyworker, I had a regular exchange with a colleague. Inside her closet, where I would hang my clothes, a large poster was on the wall. It was an enlarged photo of a chick breaking out of its shell. The caption on the bottom read: "Now what?" Hilarious and so awfully true! We are not given a set of instructions as to how to cope with being plopped into this earthly existence. Nor are we given a road map to find our way back to our origin. We have created religions as vehicles with their prescribed highways as a response to this fundamental urge.

Religion comes from the Latin *re-ligio*, which means going back to the root. Unfortunately, most religions have not worked for many of us. While the essence of their founders may have been sound, I believe that the interpretation and application of the principles often compromise their purpose. There is a problem with personifying God as a separate supernatural entity that will reward or punish us in accordance with our deeds or misdeeds. Don't get me wrong! I believe in cause and effect and what goes around comes around. I just take issue with the glaring contradiction of conceptualizing God as an external Being while proclaiming God is One. If he or she is One in the absolute sense, he or she cannot be other. He, she, or it is none other than each of us. Christianity helped bridge the gap by offering us the humanization of God in Jesus Christ. What attracted me to Buddhism was that properly understood (though that has not always been the case with some schools of Buddhism), Buddha is not a God to be worshipped or feared or devoted to outside of oneself but is our very essence. It is said that upon his enlightenment, the historical Gautama Buddha pronounced: "I alone am responsible." That means that Buddha cannot be found outside of me, and nobody else is responsible for my destiny. This does not mean that I can control everything that life presents to me any more than I can control everything that goes on inside my body or mind, with its trillions of interactions happening every second. However, it does mean that I am ultimately connected with everything and everyone, and the degree to which I am aware is the degree that I shall think, speak, and act responsibly and cause the least suffering for myself and others. As the wise verse in the Bible states: "Love thy neighbor as thyself."

Know Thyself

Who am I? Back in Chapter 2, I shared my experience at fifteen of confronting this fundamental question and how it set me on the course my life has taken. My years of dedication to meditation practice and philosophic investigation taught me a lot about how my mind worked and how awareness of its processes could help me modify my experiences to maintain a relatively stable and sane quality of life. However, the elephant in the room was that I knew I had not answered the question of who I am intellectually nor attained certifiable self-realization or enlightenment.

Albert Einstein claimed that we could not solve a problem with the same mind that created the problem.

We need to think outside of the box. Years of meditation have helped me cultivate the capacity to be aware of my thoughts and their repercussions on my body and psyche while sitting in the stable and relatively predictable sanctuary of the time and place I set aside to meditate in. Undeniably, this regular practice carried over into my experiences and interactions outside of this protected context such that I could respond with some degree of consciousness rather than react impulsively to the triggers that life presents to all of us.

However, it was evident that many of my tendencies to act or react in certain ways in certain situations or dynamics in my relationships remained unchanged, and this was not only away from the refuge of my meditation seat but even at times while meditating. In fact, my tendencies or patterns even influenced the way I meditated. I still had a lot to learn about how my mind worked. The problem was that "I" was not sufficiently aware of who "I" was at any given moment. My awareness and capacity to be a clear arbitrator were heavily conditioned by the differing and conflicting "me's" that make up my ego complex. How can I think out of the box if I am not even aware of being in a box, not to mention what is in this box called "me"?

According to legend, the aphorism *Know thyself* was carved into stone at the entrance to the temple of Apollo at Delphi in Greece. In ancient Greece, self-knowledge was valued as fundamental. They built monumental temples with statues representing the gods they honored. In Greek mythology, each god or goddess represented archetypal energies that exist as potentials in each of us. The ancient Greeks understood our universal Self and life experience as having many aspects or energies that we call upon in accordance with our needs. These timeless principles are just as relevant today as they were then. It is crucial for us to know ourselves—whether our archetypal persona or our more unique persona—if we are to have any agency in the quality of our personal, social, and professional lives. Voice Dialogue is one key to opening the doors to our inner selves.

I was introduced to the Voice Dialogue method as part of my training in Hellerwork, a structural integration process involving manipulation of myofascial tissue, movement re-education, and dialogue. Voice Dialogue is like a game of musical chairs. The facilitator sits in one chair opposite the individual being facilitated. However, in addition to the central chair opposite the facilitator, the one being facilitated has other chairs on either side or around them. The dialogue starts with the facilitated sitting in the central chair. The idea is that a different seat or position is assigned to each of the energetic patterns or subpersonalities identified during the dialogue process. The dialogue will not just be between two persons or selves but with several of the multiple selves or personas that make up the ego complex of the individual being facilitated. Each chair is the seat of a distinct energy where we don a different mask or take on a different identity.

Though other therapeutic techniques, such as psychodrama and Gestalt therapy, invoke the expression of various personas in the participants, what is unique about Voice Dialogue is that the stories expressed by our different personas and their implications in our lives are less important than sensitizing our awareness to their distinct energetics. The primary and ultimate purpose of the work is to cultivate what is called an Aware Ego in Voice Dialogue. The Aware Ego is not a self that can be identified but rather a transitory process that results from "teasing out" the various selves that make up our ego.

When we first take our seat in the central seat, the Operating Ego is sitting there. The facilitator begins a dialogue with this one, and once a few "voices" ("the part of me that...") have made themselves evident, the facilitator will ask the participant to choose a seat or position other than where they are sitting in the center to assume that identity fully. The combination of the physical displacement and the facilitator addressing that part of the individual as a distinctly different person helps the facilitator and the facilitated get to know each persona without confusing interference from other parts of the ego complex. Then the facilitator will invite the participant to return to the central seat and separate from the energetic just engaged with. It should feel as if that persona remains behind in their separate chair. The facilitator will then guide the participant to feel the difference in their body. It is as if one mask has been removed and another one behind it is accessed. This is often followed by a similar process with that persona in another seat or position, after which the participant is again directed to return to the central position and separate from that energy. Each time the participant returns to the central position, they are invited to feel the shift. It is a bit like shifting gears in the transmission of a vehicle.

Engaging in each persona is like shifting into that gear, and the neutral position is the transitory zone from which one can choose which "gear" or persona to engage with as the situation demands. Just as the neutral position is not a gear, the central position does not belong to a self or persona but to a transitory process that brings awareness to the operating ego and gradually transforms it into an Aware Ego.

Primary, Suppressed, and Repressed Selves

As mentioned earlier, we each have multiple personas. This is not to say that we all suffer from multiple personality disorder, which is a condition that results in there being no awareness of personality shifts. However, awareness is a relative thing. We are more or less aware of the personas that influence our behavior and life experience. We may feel quite stable in our identity when we are strongly identified with one persona, but the degree to which we are identified with it reflects our lack of awareness of other energies or personas within us.

How does a facilitator know which persona to work with in a Voice Dialogue session? The first answer is that the client lets the facilitator know. Though the goal of Voice Dialogue is to develop an Aware Ego, I have facilitated hundreds of clients, some of them for extended sessions, and I cannot remember one of them who came to me with that purpose as their primary motivation to work with me. I prefer to call myself a facilitator rather than a therapist in the context of Voice Dialogue because what makes this work so powerful is that it is the client or participant who is doing most of the work, so their own process empowers them.

This work is therapeutic and what it has in common with other therapies is that those who want to do it have a problem or something going on in their life that they need help dealing with. So, the dialogue begins with the facilitator asking the client why they want to do this work or, in the case of those who have already answered that question and are returning to further their education in this process, what is going on at this time in their lives. This sets in motion a dialogue, not unlike any other, between two people. However, the facilitator is responsible for listening sensitively to the story and the different energies that the client expresses and asking questions that facilitate both the facilitator and the client's becoming aware of the actors or characters in the story.

In Voice Dialogue, the focus is not so much on what happened, why it happened, or even fixing the problem. What is most important is Who is involved in the dynamic. When we are aware of our energetics in any given situation, we are in a much better position to choose how to respond. That is not always obvious because personas, the masks we wear, conceal other personas that are less evident or even thoroughly concealed or buried in our subconscious mind-body. In fact, more concealed personas are crucial in causing problems and resolving them. The less we are conscious of an energy in us, the less we have control over it and the more havoc it can create. This is where we need to introduce the concept of *primary, suppressed,* and *repressed* selves.

The *primary* selves are the personas we most identify with and recognize as "me." They are also quite evident to others as these are the selves we present to others. Over the course of our lives, we have developed these selves to survive, protect ourselves, and get what we need or want. They usually bring us to a facilitator or therapist because they are interested in solving our problems or surmounting our challenges. Some examples of primary selves are the Controller/Protector, the Pusher, the Inner Critic/Outer Judge, the Pleaser, the Responsible Father, the Nurturing Mother, the Caregiver, the Teacher/Mentor, the Entertainer, the Observer, the Vulnerable Child, the Social Butterfly, the Artist, the Victim, the Rebel, and the list goes on. There are also archetypal energies like the Warrior, the Hero, the Creator, the Jester, the Wise Sage, the Lover, the Outlaw, the Magician, etc. Of course, they are only primary if they are dominant traits that we identify with.

The same energies can be suppressed or repressed. We may be aware of a *suppressed* energy as part of who we are, but our dominant primary personas tend to suppress it because they perceive it as a threat to their agenda. A typical example is the suppression of the Vulnerable Child by a Controller/Protector or someone in the Controller/Protector team like a Pusher, Inner Critic, or Hero. Primary and suppressed personas are usually closely related in a shared dynamic. As mentioned earlier, we are born vulnerable, so one of the first personas we develop at the beginning of our lives is a Controller/Protector to protect our vulnerability. These are followed by the development of other personas with their particular dynamics.

None of the energies are inherently bad or good, but when we are identified with one more than the other, the one that is suppressed may be perceived as an enemy or at least as a nuisance, and their conflicting agendas can cause problems. This can become a more serious problem in the case of repressed energies. A *repressed* energy has been so thoroughly suppressed that we have absolutely no consciousness of that potential existing within us. In Voice Dialogue, it is referred to as a disowned self. The term is very appropriate. All our personas are our inner family of selves. As such, they need to be embraced even if they have differing characters.

We tend not to like those that are not like us. A good parent may not like their child's behavior, but they will continue to love them and, hopefully, try to understand them. Disowning a child is a tragedy when the parent has ceased to consider them a family member. The root of the problem is usually that the parent has disowned the corresponding energy in themselves, so they are incapable of understanding or empathizing with that energy in their child.

So how does one identify a disowned self or energy pattern in oneself if we have no consciousness or familiarity with it? Here is one way. Think of someone that you despise. It does not have to be someone you know. It could be a historical figure or a living person with notoriety for good or bad reasons. Write down a few characteristics of this person. Now think of a person you admire and jot down a few characteristics of this person. The characteristics you have noted are quite likely disowned in yourself. What the person you despise and the person you admire have in common is that you have distanced yourself from identifying with either one of them, and these characteristics or qualities exist in you, or else you wouldn't be triggered by them. As the expression goes, it takes one to know one. This does not mean they would express themselves the same way in you but repressing them will not be without consequences.

In analytical psychology, disowned selves are part of what is called our shadow side. People tend to be reluctant to embrace their shadow and disowned selves in particular. This is understandable, as we tend to be afraid of the unknown. Also, shadows are dark, and words like dark and shady suggest someone or something not to be trusted. We need to understand that the shadow just means that which is not exposed to the light of our conscious mind. It is just the part of us that we are not aware of. The shadow is not negative or bad. Energy is not bad or good, so there are no bad or good personas, whether they exist in our conscious or unconscious minds. Water is not bad or good in itself. The same water that serves and sustains our bodies and environment can work against us if it is dammed up and bursts its confines.

Similarly, if we ignore or neglect energies in us, they can build up and sometimes burst their confines in destructive ways that are out of our control. We can control what we are aware of but what lies outside of our awareness will affect us and influence the direction of our lives without even knowing it. The good news is that, conversely, if we can become aware of these personas and understand them as worthy of our attention, they will become our allies rather than our enemies. This will not only bring us more inner harmony but empower us to connect with others more effectively and expand our capacity to manifest what we need or want in our life.

For example, Lonny has a work colleague that is proud, arrogant, insensitive, and lacks tact in social situations. Lonny can't understand how he not only gets away with it, but his colleague just got a raise, earning more than he does. Lonny knows he is more knowledgeable and attentive to producing quality results in his tasks. Lonny is polite and reserved and careful not to say or do things that may elicit disapproval or judgment from others. He finds his colleague's way of coming across embarrassing and irritating and the very sound of his voice irks him.

Lonny identifies with a polite and cautious Pleaser, which is one of his primary personas. His colleague's brash and arrogant persona is so unlike his own. It is one of his disowned selves. The reason his colleague's behavior so triggers him is that this energy actually exists as a potential in his own psyche. Still, it has been thoroughly repressed either because he witnessed the destructive effect of this kind of behavior or personally experienced negative repercussions from being subjected to it. The theory of subpersonalities makes sense to him, so he is willing to try Voice Dialogue to help him deal with his disagreeable work environment, which has made him feel depressed and anxious over time.

Lonny describes his situation to his facilitator and expects that he will get some sympathy, support, and guidance on how to surmount the problem. Instead, the facilitator suggests that he would benefit from getting in touch with the part of him that is like the persona of his colleague at work. He cannot imagine that he has an energy like that and even resents the suggestion that he does. The facilitator explains that all these potentials exist within each of us, and how they express themselves in each of us will likely differ from the particular expression we have encountered in others. His facilitator also mentions that it is normal to feel like Lonny is playing a part that may not feel authentic at first. This is reassuring for Lonny's primary personas to hear, as the last thing he wants is to be identified with such an energy. The facilitator then asks Lonny if the proud and insensitive part of him were in the room, where he'd be sitting or standing. Lonny chooses to move his chair forward and to the left of where he was sitting in the center.

Once Lonny is settled in his new seat, the facilitator asks him to tell him about himself as the part of him that corresponds to the colleague's energy. From this position, any part of him other than the self occupying the new seat is referred to as "he" or "she" to help him dis-identify from his primary selves sitting in the central seat earlier. The facilitator then asks this part of Lonny if he has sometimes expressed himself in Lonny's life.

At first, Lonny is at a loss about who he is in this position or what to say. So, the facilitator reminds him that he is the part of Lonny that can be proud, arrogant, insensitive, and lacks tact in social situations. Lonny tries to think of when he has ever been like that and draws a blank. Then the facilitator asks if Lonny can remember when he was a young boy and experienced these characteristics. Lonny cannot remember acting like his colleague at work but remembers enjoying elementary school and getting good grades. Report cards were an exciting occasion for him, and he voiced his exuberance when he was among the first in his class. He liked the competitive aspect at the time. However, each time he showed his report card and shared his pride over his accomplishment with his father, his father would not congratulate him but say: "You can do better than that." This became increasingly discouraging to him, and by the time he got to seventh grade, his grades started to lower. Peer pressure in high school didn't help. The feedback he got was that if you did well, you were a nerd, and it wasn't cool. So, his grades were mediocre in high school, and he kept a lower profile.

The facilitator then invites Lonny to channel the elementary school version of himself when he was more expressive and proud of his accomplishments and asks him to share how this felt. Then he asked him how he feels about the way Lonny is at work and if he has anything to tell him. Without hesitation, this part of Lonny looks over to where Lonny was sitting earlier and tells him he should let his light shine and let people at work see what he can do. He was aware that a part of Lonny was concerned about being insensitive to others and felt that standing out would rub people the wrong way. However, from this position, he can confidently tell the other part of Lonny that letting his light shine didn't necessarily mean that he had to be loud and insensitive like his colleague. Not only would he not be rejected by his co-workers, but they would probably be happy for him and respect his performance. The facilitator notices that he was leaning forward and was quite animated. He asks him again how he feels, and this time, this part of Lonny rather enthusiastically responds: "I feel good!" When the facilitator asks him how this feels in his body, he says that he feels his feet firm on the ground and strong in his core. The facilitator then thanks him for sharing and asks Lonny to return to the central seat where he was sitting earlier.

As soon as Lonny resumes his seat, the facilitator asks him to imagine that the bold and animated part of him that had just expressed himself is still sitting in the space in front of him to his left and consciously separate from this energy. Then the facilitator asks him how he feels in his body now, sitting here. It takes him a little while to separate from the energy that had just filled him but eventually, he remarks that he feels less energized here but not anxious like when the dialogue session was starting. He feels calmer, though he notices his right shoulder feels a little stiff. When a new sensation like this appears, it can be an indicator that another energy has been activated by the dialogue that just took place. The facilitator asks to speak with the part of Lonny that is his usual persona at work. He asks Lonny to choose another seat from where he is sitting in the center or where he sat in the dialogue with the "let my light shine" persona. Lonny takes a seat to the right of center. Note: It is best to have extra seats already available to move to.

The facilitator then asks this part of Lonny how he feels about what the bold part of him had to say earlier. He responds that what he said makes sense, but he is a little apprehensive about putting that strategy into action at work. The facilitator asks him if he would be okay with that energy in Lonny being expressed as long as he approves of it. He agrees with this, and after a brief recap of what was shared by the other energy, he feels more comfortable. He even notices that the slight pain and stiffness in his right shoulder are no longer there. The facilitator then asks Lonny to resume his seat in the center.

This central seat is the position assigned to the Aware Ego position, but it is most of the time occupied by the operating ego, which is a confluence of several personas in our inner psychic family. The purpose of Voice Dialogue is to stimulate awareness to support the development of the Aware Ego, which is not a distinct self or persona but rather a dynamic process within which one has more freedom of choice in how one acts or responds to situations that arise in our lives.

So, at this point, the facilitator asks Lonny to imagine and feel the energy from the seat he occupied as the bold and energetic person in front of him and feel its effect in his body-mind. Then he asks him to shift his awareness to the energy he felt in the seat to his left, occupied by his more reserved and conservative persona, and feel what is happening in his body-mind. Finally, he asks him to separate from both of these energies and notice what he is feeling now. This sensibility is not always easy to access, so other techniques are also used in Voice Dialogue to facilitate this experience.

Once the individual being facilitated is back in the central position of the Aware Ego, a conversation can take place to exchange feedback, ask questions about the experience, and discuss the possible application of what has been learned in one's daily life and relationships. For example, one possible outcome of the example just provided is that Lonny will have modified his perception of his co-worker and his own tendency to keep a low-key profile at work. He may now feel more confident expressing his own talents and letting his light shine. Admittedly the example I have just shared is simpler and less dramatic than some sessions can be in this kind of work. This work is therapeutic, but I am calling it a process rather than therapy to distinguish it from other therapeutic techniques in which the therapist may be more relied upon to direct the process. In Voice Dialogue, the client is given the tools to drive his own vehicle, so to speak.

Empowerment comes from cultivating self-awareness and learning how to apply this awareness in real-life situations.

Dreamwork

Another fascinating and powerful tool that is available to all of us in our quest to know ourselves and cultivate some agency in the evolution of our lives is Dreamwork. As evidenced in the description of the development of our personalities, we are not only identified with our tangible bodies and waking life situations but also with our habitual stories and how they affect and play out in our daily lives. Ironically, we tend to regard our dreams as imaginary and irrelevant and our waking life as real and relevant, yet the course our surface-level minds carve out for us in our waking lives is determined mostly by the subliminal or unconscious energies that we have little or no awareness of.

Carl Jung said: "Who looks outside, dreams; who looks inside, awakes." He also said: "Your vision will become clear only when you can look into your own heart." To truly understand who we are and who is running the show, we need to pay attention to the messages we receive from the depths of our unconscious minds. The self we identify with in our waking lives tends to filter out the information or messages in the background of our conscious lives as irrelevant, extraneous, or trivial, yet dreams are the unconscious mind's way of bypassing the filter of our "conscious" ego-minds to try to get our attention. When we are asleep, the ego mind is off duty, so the energies hiding in the depths of our unconscious minds can emerge onto the mind screen unedited. Part of the reason we may not consider them relevant is that they often do not make sense to us since their language is in symbols. It is as if someone were to address us in a foreign language, and because we do not understand, we would not consider what they are telling us to be relevant. That could pose a problem in certain situations where the information might be crucial.

One could fairly ask why dreams use the language of symbols rather than the literal language we use in our waking state. The more fundamental question is, what purpose do dreams serve? It is commonly accepted that when we are sleeping, the body gets a chance to rest from its usual functions of locomotion, eating and digesting, and the multiple activities we fill our day with. During this time, the body's energies are given the opportunity to clean, repair, and regenerate our complex network of systems. Similarly, it is thought that dreams are the way the mind processes the experiences that it has recorded in its memory bank during our daily waking activities, both in the time immediately preceding and accumulated or built up in the preceding days. However, when we speak of memory, *whose* memory are we talking about? As evidenced in the process of Voice Dialogue, each persona has its own distinct perception of itself and the world it experiences. Each persona also has its own distinct memory. As we have seen in the description of the Voice Dialogue process, the perceptions and memories we are aware of are those of the dominant persona that we are most identified with. Concealed behind these masks are different points of view and wisdom that we are not accessing. This limits our capacity to "think outside of the box" of our habitual grooves. As a result, we limit our ability to solve problems, resolve inner and outer conflicts, and manifest our full creative potential. Dreams are our built-in mechanism for our unconscious potential to penetrate the veil of our primary persona and reveal to us valuable information to reflect on our lives with more clarity and guide us in our choices.

For our dreams to evade the editing or censoring of our dominant ego-mind, they are presented to us in symbolic language. The people and things in our internal movies are symbolic representations of energetics at play within our own psyche. Even if we dream of actual people, things, or events we know or situations that we have experienced, which may have something to do with our dream's content, dreams are not just the regurgitation of our life experiences. The unconscious mind is a storehouse of knowledge of every impression that has been engraved in our mind and body, whether we are aware of them or not, and has the uncanny ability to call up just what we need to know at a particular moment that we would not otherwise likely discover with our conscious mind. It does not just replay a scenario that represents our current or past experience. It can also predict the direction our situation may evolve into. To interpret and understand the message of our dreams, we need to decipher the code it presents to us.

Though there are many dream dictionaries that provide interpretations of common dream symbols, and they can certainly be useful, each of us is unique and what symbols represent to each of us is personal so the ideal person to interpret the symbols of our dreams is ourselves. Though dreams can provide a perspective and direction for outer situations, they are also a portal to the innermost workings of our mind, so it is well worth the effort to pay attention to their personal message for us. Decoding and interpreting our dreams requires some practice and a little more time in the beginning until we are more used to it, but the method is relatively simple.

Here is the method I have been using for years. First, for those of you who may think that you don't dream, we all dream but may not remember what we dreamt or even that we had a dream. For those who don't remember their dreams, the good news is that we can train the mind to remember. Before going to sleep at night, simply ask your mind to remember your dreams. Don't underestimate the power of intention. You may not remember your dreams the first few nights, but eventually, you will. It is also important to know that you don't need to remember all your dreams or even all of one dream to benefit from this practice. Just record whatever you remember, and don't concern yourself with telling it in order. Just write or speak whatever comes to your mind, and your mind will likely fill in the blanks as you get into the flow. Don't worry about "getting it right." What you recall and what you dreamt come from the same source. Do this as soon as you can upon awakening, as your waking state mind will erase it from your memory if you wait too long. Relieve yourself in the bathroom if necessary but if you wait until you have prepared a coffee, or worse, check notifications on your phone, you will be surprised how quickly you can completely forget even what seem to be memorable dreams.

I review the dream in my mind while I am still lying in bed with my eyes closed because this allows me to not only imprint the dream in my surface-level memory but also to remain in the mood of the dream, which is also relevant to its message for me. The one who experienced the dream remembers it best, which is not the same self operating in most of our waking life.

Record your dream either orally into a recorder or in writing, whichever medium allows you to do so without too much reflection. I am used to free flow writing from my practice of Morning Pages, which will be described later, so I choose to write it out, which allows me to easily refer to the written text for the following process of extracting the symbols.

Once you have recorded your dream, take a sheet of paper in your dream journal or a writing app on your computer, if you prefer, and divide your page with a line down the middle. In the left-hand column, list the symbols in your dream. Include every person, animal, object, place, and event, including you, the dreamer. Then, in the right-hand column, write just a few words to describe the quality or characteristic of each person or thing in the left column beside the symbol. You are describing an energetic for each symbol as it manifested in your dream, so if, for example, a colleague at work was in your dream, they may embody a particular energy in your experience with them at work, but they express different behavior in your dream. The combination of their usual character and the variation in the dream is relevant in this analysis. Also, you, the dreamer, will be expressing a particular energy in your inner family of selves, such as an observer energy, a maternal or paternal energy, a playful or mischievous child energy, etc. A lifeguard tower in your dream might symbolize a position of responsibility for others' safety, but if it is empty or filled with toys, it will, of course, symbolize quite a different dynamic. Describe this with as few words as possible.

The next step is to retell your dream using the de-coded qualities, characteristics, or dynamics as a representation of a part of yourself. Even if you dreamt of actual people you know and have interacted with recently, in the context of your dream as the medium your unconscious mind is using to communicate with you, it is not about someone else; it is about how the parts of yourself— your inner family of selves—are interacting within you and affecting your daily life experience. So, for example, you will write: "The responsible father in me was concerned about the care-free childlike parts of me not paying attention to a rising tide of unknown and powerful currents threatening the easy-going atmosphere of ...etc." It will sound awkward and cumbersome to retell the story of your dream in this way and probably sound less entertaining than the literal story of your dream but trust the process, as the next step will reveal what your universal mind wants you to know.

Finally, read what you have just written or listen to what you have recorded. At first, it may not make much sense, but if you receive the information and allow it to impress itself in your mind, your mind will take care of the rest. Think about how it may address what has been happening in your life recently, whether in actual events and relationships or in your thoughts and feelings. You may be tempted to omit some object symbols thinking that they are insignificant or too complicated to interpret as a part of yourself or unrelated to your analysis of the dream, but I have often found that they can contain the most insightful perspectives once deciphered. Trust the process.

Interpreting your dreams is like consulting an oracle or a psychic. The revelations ring true because they resonate with or expose what we already know inside but may ignore because our dominant personas may not want to deal with knowledge that threatens their agenda, modus operandi, or self-mage. A clairvoyant can penetrate the filters of our protective persona because they can be a more objective observer, not burdened by our subjective identifications. Of course, clairvoyants have their own personalities and identifications, so it is not always easy to trust what they are telling us. The advantage of self-readings through Dreamwork is that there is no one else to trust or mistrust. One can only trust someone else if one trusts one's own discernment.

Cultivating the art of Dreamwork is a fascinating and empowering tool for self-knowledge and personal growth. Some are endowed with the capacity to consult inner guides. I am not aware of mine, if I have any, but I have often had the feeling after interpreting a dream that a higher power knows me intimately and brilliantly and lovingly lets me know that I am never alone. That is a precious experience!

Combining Voice Dialogue with Dreamwork

Voice Dialogue and Dreamwork can make a powerful pair. You can recount your dream to a Voice Dialogue facilitator, and your facilitator can ask you to assume the seat of one or more energetics in your dream and personify that part of your dream experience. It does not have to be a person; it could be an animal or an inanimate object. If this part of you had a voice, what would it say? You might be surprised! Say I become Daryl's car in his dream. The facilitator gets me into character and then asks me what my role is in his life and how it is going. I might respond with: "I am his vehicle for getting to where he wants to go. How's it going? Hmm, well, he could check my tire pressure and look under the hood more often, and I would be able to serve him better." This might make me more aware of how I have been identified with getting things done and "going places" and not giving enough attention to my psychic or physical health. One may not need to dialogue with every symbol in the dream as their significance may be revealed in the dialogue with just a few of them.

Active Imagination

Active Imagination is an alternative to Voice Dialogue for giving voice to unconscious currents in the storehouse of our psyche. Developed by Carl Jung, it resembles Sigmund Freud's method of free associations. In the latter, the subject is invited to speak freely about anything that crosses their mind without concern about being logical or politically correct. The difference with Active Imagination is that one focuses on images and visualizations rather than words, so the experience is like a waking dream. The goal is to live the image and its associated emotions, in other words, to evoke its essence. The purpose of this exercise is not only to analyze the significance of the image, visualization, or dream content intellectually but to connect with it intimately and thereby facilitate its message traversing the threshold between our unconscious and conscious mind. The degree to which we can feel its essence like lifeblood flowing through our body-mind is the degree to which we can benefit from the therapeutic power of this work. When we allow ourselves to live the fantasy in this way, we can better appreciate why Jung claimed: "Who looks outside, dreams; who looks inside, awakes."

One application of Active Imagination is to use the content of one's dreams in a similar way to what was described previously in the context of a Voice Dialogue process. However, instead of engaging the energy of the imagination in a dialogue with an external facilitator, one can engage directly with the energy oneself. For example, let's say that a grizzly bear has popped up in my imaginary world, whether in dream sleep, a daydream, or some other context that is calling for my attention. I can use my imagination to become the bear and act out its energy. The bear may have something to say, but words are not necessary here.

The important thing is to feel the energy of the bear. As with Dreamwork, what the bear energy conveys depends on the context in which it has emerged. For example, if it is a mama bear with her cubs, it may be quite different from a male bear or a bear cub. Once I have lived or embodied its energy, I can change roles and interact with the bear. I can simply approach and pet it or stand in front of where it manifested earlier and ask what it wants me to know. Even if the bear first appeared in the context of a dream, I do not need to communicate with it in accordance with the content of the story of the dream. As a persona in my psyche, it has a life of its own, not restricted to the context in which it manifested itself to me. Then I wait for its response to appear in my imagination. There is no right or wrong response. It's all just as real as I, the imaginer, is.

I used to be quite skeptical about my capacity to visualize and benefit from any practice that involved such methods. Though part of my practice as a Buddhist monastic involved Tibetan Buddhist visualizations, I had never felt that I was doing it "right." Part of the problem was that I had heard that visualizations could be more "real" than what our eyes see in our waking state. One can wax philosophically at length about what constitutes reality, but a few experiences I had after leaving monastic life convinced me that what I had considered inauthentic visualizations deserved my attention.

Part of my training as a massage therapist required me to participate in a guided group visualization at the end of the morning session. I tended to "space out" during the detailed description that was meant to guide us into our inner knowing hidden in the depths of our psyche. I would drift off into a reverie that basically felt like I had fallen asleep or at least lapsed into a daydream and missed much of what I was supposed to visualize.

At the end of the session, each of us was asked to share our experiences. When it was my turn, I was not shy to admit that it had not worked for me as I had disconnected and missed most of what was said. I had come to accept that this was just one faculty I did not seem to possess. The instructor asked me what I had experienced even if I didn't remember the images she had presented. I replied that I imagined different things but was unable to visualize. She asked me to share some of what I imagined. I shared the images that I saw, and this took several minutes. At the end of my sharing, she commented that for someone who is not good at visualizing, I certainly had a lot of imagination. She pointed out that I had shared more images than anyone else in the group shared.

Mildly encouraged, I went home. When I arrived, I noticed an envelope in my mailbox with a see-through window that revealed a yellow document. I don't remember the physical sensation I felt, but it was probably a shiver up my spine. My mailman usually came at about one in the afternoon, and I had seen that envelope as one of the images during the guided visualization that took place at around the same time. This turned out to be my first unemployment cheque, so I would not have known that it would be yellow and in an envelope with a transparent window. The next time I did the guided visualization with my massage class, I "imagined" a conflict in the kitchen of the restaurant that was part of a New Age bookstore, health food store, and restaurant, where I had worked as manager of the bookstore until it was closed down. My friend Stefan was still working there, so later, when I got home, I asked him if he had been involved in a conflict. He hadn't, but he had witnessed an argument between the chef and one of his staff in the kitchen. These two experiences, in close succession, impressed themselves in my memory and helped me learn to validate what I had considered irrelevant or trivial thoughts or images.

Yes, thoughts can also be worthy of our attention. Years later, I was involved in a guided group regression as a part of my training as a Voice Dialogue practitioner in California. I had experienced the same tendency to "space out" during the session and when it was time to ask my wisdom voice inside what I had come to learn in this life, what came to mind was that I was born an identical twin, so I considered that I had come to learn about duality, which is ironic considering how much I have been focused on cultivating the vision of oneness.

I hesitated to accept this answer as an authentic response from my wisdom voice because it seemed more like a thought creation than a voice speaking to me. Witnessing this self-doubt, I realized that this voice came from my inner critic. I thanked it for sharing and gratefully received the insight from my wisdom voice.

These experiences taught me that our expectations are conditioned by our dominant identifications and can act as roadblocks in our evolution. Whatever faculty I wish to develop will only be enhanced by giving credit to how it manifests in my unique experience.

Morning Pages

Pioneered by the writer Julia Cameron in her book *The Artist's Way*, Morning Pages is a powerful tool for releasing one from the chains of writer's block and enhancing creativity in general. It is also a powerful medium for accessing the potentials hidden in the depths of our unconscious mind-body. I am using the term mind-body because the mind and all the impressions it has accumulated permeate every cell of our body-mind. Most of our body experiences happen without our awareness and, therefore, in the realm of the unconscious, yet it is crucial to our survival and functionality.

We use speech to express our thoughts to others, but it also mirrors what is going on in our minds. Even when we think, before uttering what we think, we use words to process and organize our thoughts. Thus, speech is an important tool in the chest of our internal editor. When we write, as I'm doing right now, the editor has even more opportunities to filter what is appropriate or not to express. The question is appropriate for who? Most of the time, thinking before we speak affords us more possibility of communicating in ways that work for us to get along with others and get our needs met. What is appropriate in this context is determined by our dominant persona that we have developed for surviving and managing our daily lives.

However, when it comes to the inner work of digging for the gold that lies within the rich storehouse of our unconscious mind, we need to throw caution to the wind to liberate the flow of treasures that not only nourish creativity but can also provide insights to guide us in how we navigate our existence.

The idea of Morning Pages is that we should not lift our pen from the page to pause and reflect but rather keep writing whatever comes to mind without concern about it being logical or intelligent. We are not writing for anyone else but ourselves. No one will ever see it unless we choose to share a selection. It is like a private journal. It is to be done first thing in the morning before the waking mind kicks in to censor what we write. Because dream interpretation also needs to be done soon after arising, I allow myself to sometimes start that process at the beginning of my Morning Pages. After all, they do share the same source. However, the pure experience of Morning Pages is to write with no purpose.

The length is approximately 750 words (2 or 3 pages, depending on the size of your pages and letters). It is to be done in cursive so that the letters flow into each other, so put aside your keyboard. A friend of mine chooses to speak into his phone recorder. I wouldn't do that because I have found that my mind has more opportunities to pause, reflect, and be self-conscious when speaking out loud. The moving hand seems to entrain the mind to stay in the flow. Your inner critic may get a little antsy when it witnesses the gibberish that makes its way onto your page. That is your cue to put that persona aside and continue. Don't be surprised if, soon after that, you will perceive relevant insights and wisdom in the stream of thoughts.

Then another persona like your Pusher-Achiever, your Teacher or Attention-Getter persona will seize the opportunity and want to appropriate those gems of wisdom. Letting that one go as well brings you back to the present moment. This is a discipline with a beginning and an end. The process takes 30 to 40 minutes, but it makes more time in terms of how it clarifies your thoughts and aligns them with what is more crucial for the evolution of your life. If you need to get up earlier to make time for this practice, you will find that the energy saved by freeing your mind from the chains of limiting habit patterns will make up for it. It will also enhance your productivity and increase your self-confidence. If you want to learn more about this technique and related techniques, check out Julia Cameron's book, *The Artist's Way*. [23]

The Shadow

I cannot conclude this chapter on inner work without a few words about the shadow. The shadow or "shadow self" (which is misleading as there are many selves with our shadow) is a central concept in Jungian psychology. It refers to the unknown or "dark" side of our personality or inner psychic family of selves. It contains instinctive and irrational energies that we are completely unaware of yet profoundly influence our lives.

For many, shadow work is intimidating or unwelcome because it implies negative and socially unacceptable characteristics.

"Dark" suggests gloomy, dire, dreadful, and dangerous. Actually, the shadow is simply the side of us that does not see the light of day. The definition of a shadow is a dark area where an opaque object blocks light from a light source. It is the primary selves of our ego complex that create our shadow. Interestingly, the shadow of an object is usually larger than the object that casts the shadow. Our psychic shadow is also larger than the primary personality that we are aware of and that others see. I have mentioned earlier how the mind can be compared to an ocean where the surface represents the waking or conscious mind, and what lies beneath

---

[23] *The Artist's Way: A Spiritual Path to Higher Creativity* by Julia Cameron; Profile 2020

the surface represents our unconscious mind, which is far vaster.

It is also a lot darker down there. Perhaps this contributes to the fear factor. The two-dimensional cross-section of a shadow we call a silhouette is a reverse projection of the object blocking the light. Our psychic shadow is exactly that. It is the other side of the aspect of our self that we identify with and show to others. The shadow contains the unconscious parts of our personality that our conscious ego doesn't want to identify in itself.

You may recall that at the beginning of this section, I asked the question: Why would we want to explore this area of ourselves? Well, we know that what we are not aware of, we have no control over and what we have no control over is likely to have control over us. However, it goes beyond controlling our own behavior.

The energies that we repress within will project themselves into our conscious lives. They will manifest in the kind of people we attract and the situations we attract or are unconsciously attracted to. Psychological projection happens when we project a characteristic we are unaware of in ourselves onto someone else. Often that is not a favorable one, so the last thing our conscious ego wants to hear is that what triggers us in someone else is an aspect of ourselves that we have repressed. Whatever behaviors or attitudes we have consciously suppressed, we might have some awareness of, but when it has been repressed or thoroughly disowned, we cannot imagine that we have it in us.

So how can we know if a characteristic or energetic is a part of who we are? The first answer is that our universal self beyond the ego self-identification is everything, so nothing is excluded. There would not be good within us without there also being evil.

The second and more verifiable answer is that if you are triggered by a particular type of person or characteristic, you surely have it as well. There is a saying that a friend of mine uses: "If you spot it, you got it." I don't know who first coined this, but the idea is ancient. The ancient Greek philosopher, Epictetus, said: "When you are offended at any man's faults, turn to yourself and study your own faults."

While it may not be very encouraging to hear that what we perceive as undesirable in others lies within us, this truth can be a very positive and empowering one. First, let me clarify that if a murderer triggers you, that doesn't necessarily mean you are a murderer. When you begin the exploration of this potential within you, the work will involve discovering the characteristics of a murderer and when and where you have experienced and expressed such characteristics.

Furthermore, when you connect with that part of yourself, you will not only discover that the way it manifests in you is unique and particular to your mix of personas, but it will also typically have a positive and empowering effect. Energy that is suppressed or repressed becomes destructive. What we don't own owns us. However, when we connect with it consciously, we can harness its potential to serve us. In her book

The Dark Side of Light Chasers, Debbie Ford states that when you dig into your shadow, you will find gold.[24] The example I provided earlier of the Voice Dialogue session with Lonny in which he was introduced to the persona he had disowned, which was projected in the arrogant and aggressive behavior of one of his colleagues at work, shows how getting in touch with this energy within himself could both transform his perception of his co-worker and empower him to express more of his own potential.

When we judge another person, we reduce them to their role in the story or movie we are watching or experiencing. A good actor can have us loving them in one movie and hating them in another in which they portray a despicable character. The movies that impress me most are those in which the characters are not black and white. You find yourself despising them in one part of the movie and then empathizing with them in another. This is truer to life. When we can appreciate and understand that who we think we are or others are is influenced by the roles we have become identified with, the path of healing and transformation can begin. As Shakespeare wisely wrote in *As You Like It*: "All the world's a stage, and all the men and women are merely players."

The process of inner work and exploring our shadow requires us to think out of the box about the story of our life, our role in it, and where we want it to go. Psychology

---

[24] *The Dark Side of Light Chasers* by Debbie Ford; Riverhead Books 2010

is a young science, and it is only recently that therapy is considered a tool for self-development rather than a last resort to fix something that has gone wrong. Of course, things go wrong, and that often brings us to consult a doctor, massage therapist, psychotherapist, or other health professional or healer. The problem is that as long as things seem to be going according to plan and we are feeling relatively comfortable in our bodies, minds, and familiar routines, we don't feel a need to change anything.

What remains in the shadow will eventually break through, and things will "go wrong," whether emotionally, physically, relationally, or in our situation. By that time, we need someone else to help us "fix" what has gone wrong. Ancient Chinese doctors were paid a retainer to keep their patients healthy. If a patient got sick, the doctor would not be paid by that person until he or she got well. The message here is that the primary role of doctors and health practitioners, in general, should be to educate their patients on how to take responsibility for their mental, emotional, and physical health. We need to listen to our bodies to tap into the wisdom of this miraculous organism and heed the signs it provides us with to get our attention.

Similarly, when we find ourselves reacting in our relationships or certain situations or even struggling with inner conflicts, we need to look within instead of judging or looking to fix what seems to be outside of us. When we shine the light of our awareness into the hidden crevices of our secret inner cave, it is not so much to find a solution to a problem to change it as it is to allow ourselves to view things from another perspective and *be* changed or transformed. The more parts of ourselves we can claim into our full Me, the more whole we shall be, and the more harmonious our lives will become. If we want to improve our relationships and the world we live in, we need to start with an intimate connection with ourselves—all of them. When Buddha pronounced upon his Enlightenment: "I alone am responsible," he recognized that, ultimately, we are the author of our story.

8
Outer Work

The paradox of the universe is that it is full of duality. The last section focused on the inner work required to live a harmonious and fulfilling life. While outer work sounds like its opposite, as relativity would have it, they are mutually interdependent. We cannot have the leisure even to contemplate the practices that focus on our own body and mind if the environment that sustains us becomes toxic or barren or if we are in conflict with our brothers and sisters on this planet. Similarly, we cannot effectively sustain the health of our environment or know how to relate harmoniously with others without understanding how our own body and mind function and taking responsibility for our personal mental, emotional, and physical health.

Unfortunately, the current state of affairs is that our environment is in a headlong plunge towards disaster, at least for its human inhabitants, with global warming, air, water, and soil pollution, desertification, flooding, and degradation of elements essential for our health and survival. This is a grim picture, and according to some scientists, the situation is irreversible. My Buddhist training has taught me that suffering is part of life, but we are not powerless to deal with it. Everything has a beginning and an end, including the world we live in, but while we are here, we can do our best to make it better, not just for our progeny going forward but for ourselves right now. The fact that most of us do not put our money where our mouth is when it comes to doing our part to stop consuming products that pollute directly or indirectly or participate in polluting activities is evidence that we are under the illusion that it is not affecting us yet enough to be more concerned.

Just as we have banished parts of ourselves to our shadow, we have distanced ourselves from the reality surrounding us. Just as we are more influenced and less in control of what we are not conscious of in our psyche, the same holds true for the extension of ourselves that we call our environment. Sooner or later, we shall need to step up to the plate and face the reality that Adam and Eve's first job was to care for the garden of Eden. This does not mean that taking up gardening will solve all our problems, but it does mean that artfully living the vision of Oneness requires us to be aware of our interdependence with our environment, our connection with our fellow humans and all creatures and to educate ourselves in how to co-create with the universe.

Environmental Consciousness

I am not an environmental scientist, so this chapter will not go into detailed descriptions of what is happening to our physical environment nor the multiple technologies that are being developed to help slow down its destruction and restore it. This information is available for those who care to look for it, but the first step is awareness of the problem.

As with most destructive processes, the fundamental problem is the disconnect with the other. From an absolute perspective, we are all connected, and destruction is a part of the mix. Hinduism presents God as a trinity: Brahma, the creator aspect, represented by earth; Vishnu, the preserver/sustainer, represented by water; and Shiva, the destroyer/transformer, represented by fire. These three Gods represent the cyclical nature of our existence from birth, sustaining our life, and destruction to subsequent regeneration. From this perspective, the world we live in and our existence as a species are subject to the winds of change, just as any other natural phenomenon. Looking at the larger picture, it is hard to draw the line between what is natural and unnatural in the tragic environmental crisis we are experiencing. Nothing is permanent, and nature is always changing. However, the will to survive and not suffer is also a part of our nature. On the relative plane of our existence, we have the potential to make choices that can help sustain the environment we depend on and minimize suffering for ourselves and others. I dare say that as stewards of the garden we were born into, we are responsible for making those choices. Karma is also a part of Hindu and yogic teaching. When one understands that we are all fundamentally responsible, karma does not mean that some external force rewards or punishes us for our deeds or misdeeds. Karma is simply the reality that every cause has an effect no matter how far or close in time or place or how large or tiny the thought, speech, or action. Of course, we cannot control the infinite web of causes and effects, but how we manage our sphere of existence will certainly affect our life experience and contribute constructively or destructively to the world we live in.

No one knows the ending to the movie of our life that we are co-creating. In fact, it has no end. Life goes on. The characters in it have an ending but not the movie. We are strongly identified with the part we play and tend to focus most of our attention on our needs or wants at the exclusion of the bigger picture. We hold on to life, or rather our part in it as if we want it to be permanent, yet we know it is temporary. Ironically, our desperation to secure and add to our status is proportional to our denial of this fact. It is not our body that is afraid to die; it is the ego that is identified with it, the character we have co-created, and the part we are playing in this movie of life. The fundamental disconnect is the illusion that we are just this ego-creation, separate from others and the world we live in.

In the previous section on inner work, we saw the importance of embracing the parts of ourselves that we have denied or disowned to manifest our full potential and connect with others with more understanding. Connecting with ourselves is also essential for us to understand our connection with the world we live in. Viewing the world around us with the perspective that we have something to do with what appears to be outside of us is necessary to heal our wounded planet. The problem is that most of us are caught up in the trance of our comfortable identity and its projections, and this short-range vision limits our awareness to an intellectual abstraction. It is not much more real than a story on Google news or a Facebook post. Unfortunately, many of those in positions of power politically or financially got there because of an ego-centered vision that focuses more on short-term accomplishments than a comprehensive and sustainable approach that is good for everyone for a long time rather than a few for a short time.

Put simply, if I throw my non-biodegradable waste over the fence into my neighbor's land, even if no one is living there, it will eventually overflow into my own propertyand/or pollute the air I breathe and the water I drink. For example, I am fortunate to live within walking distance of a beautiful surfing beach in Costa Rica. The area has become very popular, so many people visit and choose to live there. Every residence needs a septic system, and unfortunately, many of them are inadequate, to say the least. The closed systems need to be emptied regularly to prevent contamination of local soil and water, but the better option is to have a system that breaks down the waste so that the remaining liquid run-off is clean, and the solid waste is minimized, thus requiring less frequent disposal. Unfortunately, many people are not following these procedures, and some of the septic disposal companies are dumping the waste into the local river. The result is that the river is polluted, and the waste has found its way to the once pristine waters of the beach. During the rainy season, it is visible and smellable in the ocean water, where we swim and surf. The lack of proper septic systems is not new in the local communities, but it has reached a level of toxicity that is now a serious concern. One might think this is a third-world issue where people lack education or more civilized infrastructures, and the government is not enforcing proper building regulations. Certainly, those are some reasons, but the truth is that lack of environmental awareness and responsibility is a problem in first-world societies as well.

Beneath the veneer of our "civilized" societies is rampant toxicity affecting our health, even if we are unaware of it. We live in our tidy boxes with relatively well-functioning systems that insulate us from the effects of our lifestyles on our surrounding environment, so most of us have only vague awareness of the current degradation of our environment, not to mention what is coming down the line. We may read or hear about it here and there in the news, but it feels quite external to our daily reality. We might cooperate with some initiatives, like separating our recyclables and compost from other waste, but do we really know what happens with all that stuff? More fundamentally, how many of us are willing to take a close look at how our lifestyles—the things we buy and the activities we engage in—impact the world we live in?

What is the solution to the fundamental problem of being disconnected from others and our environment?

The consequence of this disconnect is short-range thinking, which is a serious problem in the economics and politics of the "developed" world. The antidote to the destructiveness of short-term thinking is sustainable thinking and development. Sustainable development is development that meets the needs of the present without compromising the ability of future generations to meet their own needs.

Using recycled materials or renewable resources when building is an example of sustainable development. Large corporations are rarely interested in sustainable development because their primary goal is growth, not being sustainable. Of course, it is quite logical that sooner or later, growth will only help you if you are sustainable. However, the problem with corporations is that most of them are backed by shareholders who invest in them only so long as their shares keep growing. So, unlike humans and animals, the corporate monster never stops growing, and it has a voracious appetite. Intelligent and well-informed economists and environmentalists have made it clear that good ecology makes for a sustainable economy and that good economics is good for sustainable ecology. However, the pressures of trying to satisfy the insatiable appetite of the corporate machine impel both the corporations and the government leaders or the parties they represent that depend on the "success" of their economic record to be re-elected to favor quick gains over long-term strategies.

With the accumulation of wealth and power comes the desire to protect what has been gained. In Buddhist teaching, a central tenet is that life entails suffering, and this is symbolically illustrated by the Bhavacakra—the Wheel of Life—that represents the cycle of life, death, rebirth, and suffering that they seek to escape altogether. What we call the rat race is a version of that. Instead of a rat running interminably in a wheel cage, the Wheel of Life has three animals chasing each other's tail in the wheel's hub: a pig, a rooster, and a snake. They represent the three poisons of ignorance, attachment, and aversion that generate the cycles of cause and effect that the Buddhists call karma.

A Buddhist teacher of mine once gave a public talk to introduce lay members of our community to this concept. I was asked to illustrate each segment of a story he told on a white board. He described how a young couple wanted to build a house, so they both got jobs and saved enough money to buy some land to build on. I drew a simple picture of a piece of land with some trees and a small pond surrounded by flowers and shrubs. Then they built a small house. I added that to the picture. As time passed, the house became larger to accommodate their children, and they got a larger, more expensive car and more possessions, which were added to the picture. A wall had to be added surrounding the property to protect their possessions. In the beginning, they could dispose of their waste on the land surrounding their house, but that soon became a problem, so they threw it over the wall. This became a problem when a family bought the adjacent property. Relations with their neighbors worsened as time passed, so I was asked to add higher walls and some weaponry to protect their property. The situation escalated, and the neighbors began to build up an arsenal in reaction. Eventually, they each had a nuclear defense system to protect their holdings. The fear of losing increased in proportion to how much they had, and the more they had, the less they could enjoy it. This story sounds almost comical in its apparent exaggeration, but when it was told, we were experiencing the emotional atmosphere of the cold war between the USSR and North America, where each side lived in fear or paranoia of the possibility of someone pressing the big red button. This illustration of how short-range thinking of accumulation of comforts, possessions, and territory could result in such animosity and conflict gave us a glimpse into the root of the problem: short-range thinking based on a lack of connection with others and our environment.

As I write this, many years later, the main headline in the news is the Russian invasion of Ukraine. The war is hotter because people are being killed, but the problem is the same. Each side views the other as a threat and, of course, the evil aggressor that must be defeated. Without going into all the details, an examination of the history of this situation reveals that, despite how the media presents the scenario, both the east and west have created this conflict because of their history of wanting to extend and protect their empires. When we become identified with the extensions or projections of ourselves—our family, our tribe, our nation—and lose our awareness and connection with our essence and our oneness with all of humanity and nature, we find ourselves thrown into the insane delusion of wanting to win wars rather than understanding each other.

Plant Medicine

The section on inner work focused on how we connect with different parts of ourselves to bring more harmony into our lives and relationships with others and the environment. It also works the other way around. Our environment is also an important resource for helping us connect with ourselves so that we can live more fully, love life more, and love more.

Nature nurtures. Though I appreciate big cities for their convenience, architecture, efficient systems, infrastructures, technologies, comforts, entertainment, etc., I notice that whenever I've been away from nature for a while, I feel the difference when I return to an environment where I can spend time outside with nature. I used to notice it when I stepped out of the car upon arriving at my country cottage outside Montreal, and since living in Costa Rica near the ocean for the last several years, I notice how energized I become very soon after arriving after traveling abroad.

At my age, I am especially conscious of conserving and enhancing my energy level, so even though I spend a lot of time outdoors in this tropical paradise, if I spend a lot of time in front of a computer screen, I notice an energy drain. To counteract that effect, I work standing most of the time, which keeps me more grounded and allows more energy to flow in me. I walk around every now and then and look at the green foliage around me and the blue sky, and I feel the breeze, and listen to the sounds of the jungle. I also walk barefoot down to our beautiful beach once or twice a day, usually early morning and late afternoon, and whether it is to surf, swim, exercise, walk or even sit and watch the waves and surfers or the sunset, I feel revitalized and inspired.

Multiple scientific studies have shown that spending time outside in nature benefits physical and mental health. Just taking in the green hues of foliage and the blue of water, breathing the ion-rich air in the mountains or around moving water, hearing the sounds of nature and being inspired by the beauty of nature stimulates our hormonal system to enhance our vitality, brighten our mood, and bring more clarity to mental functions, not only for productivity but also to expand our creativity. While reading literature on this subject might motivate you to believe it, there is nothing more convincing than to experience it and nothing to lose by trying it.

Environmental consciousness is not just about being more aware or conscious of our environment. Certainly, that is an important factor in helping us connect with it and cooperate with it symbiotically. However, as a result of separating ourselves from nature, we "civilized" people have assumed that we are the only conscious or sentient beings. While it could be argued that we may have exclusivity in terms of having a self-conscious ego, we are certainly not the only creatures that feel. In fact, much of creation that we consider inanimate is more sensitive than we are. It has been demonstrated that water has feelings or at least is affected by our feelings and intentions. This phenomenon was made popular by Dr. Maseru Emoto of Japan, who conducted experiments showing how our emotions and intentions altered the crystalline structure of water and that water infused with positive intentions has positive effects on our health and vice versa when it is infused with negative intentions. Though he had his detractors and was considered by some as a "fringe" scientist, his claims were confirmed by a double-blind test of the effects of distant intention on water crystal formation published by the National Center for Biotechnology Information in 2006 [25]. The idea that nature—not just water but trees, plants, and even rocks— is animate and influences us is not new to indigenous cultures worldwide. "Civilized" cultures have labeled these cultures and their beliefs "primitive." I would agree but not in the derogatory sense. Primitive for me implies our being rooted in our original primeval connection with nature.

Hippocrates, considered the father of modern medicine, said: "Let food be your medicine." We have more or less followed this advice in the almost 2500 years since he uttered these words both in terms of appreciating the importance of proper nutrition to keep us healthy and supplementing our diet with natural and synthesized products from nature to treat particular conditions. Though it can be argued that many of our pharmaceutical medicines are derived from natural substances or plants, we have deviated from the essence of his advice by altering the original nature of our foods

---

[25] https://pubmed.ncbi.nlm.nih.gov/16979104/

through practices designed to increase production and profit and fight off interference from natural pests, and this has compromised the integrity and wholesomeness of our food sources. This has also created a consequent need for remedies to help us compensate for our lack of nutrients and attempt to cure the resulting diseases or alleviate their symptoms. Being the utilitarian creatures that we are, we have also developed impressive technology—sophisticated diagnostic and surgical tools and techniques and drugs—for dealing with the effects of our compromised connection with nature.

This should not come as any surprise as, being the ego-centered creatures that we are, we have sought to dominate our environment and all other creatures sharing it, and the way we have managed to do that is through our brilliant capacity to make tools.

Unfortunately, our reliance on tools has separated us from nature, and their production is destroying our environment. The industrial age ushered in a huge polluting impact on our environment. Manpower needed to be replaced by other energy sources to power machinery, vehicles, planes, etc.

Unfortunately, short-range thinking led us to choose toxic fuels like oil, which not only pollutes but is the resource for which the wars are being waged. It also ushered in mass farming methods and the resulting degradation of our soil, and the foods grown in it.

What does plant medicine have to do with our compromised connection with nature and each other?

As I consider describing the connection, the image that comes to mind is the Garden of Eden. I am not a biblical scholar, and even if I were, I would not likely presume to know the story's original version or its intended message. So, I won't focus on its history but rather on my sense of what it represents metaphorically. I believe that Adam and Eve represent the beginning of the human species and that their eating of the forbidden fruit of the Tree of Knowledge represents the birth of the ego or individuality.

This act separated us from God's will or universal will and gave us a sense of having independent free will—the capacity to choose good or evil. This act can be considered the original sin in that it was in disobedience of God's command not to eat of the Tree of Knowledge, but the omnipotent God, the universe, the natural order of things, whatever you would like to call it, allowed it. Oneness being comprehensive necessarily includes duality or otherness. Of course, it can be argued that animals, too, have a sense of being separate, or they wouldn't be fighting or avoiding each other and us to survive.

However, as Adam and Eve's covering their privates with a fig leaf represents, our self-consciousness has distanced us further from the natural order of things such that while we may appreciate and value Mother Nature, we tend to perceive it as outside of us, as our "environment." This word comes from the French word environ, which means around, so the environment is that which surrounds us. However, nature is not just around us; it is within and without. We perceive nature as outside of us because our individual knowledge is partial. The approach of allopathic medicine, which is predominant in the western world, is to treat symptoms and diseases using surgery, radiation, or drugs having opposite effects to the symptoms. Holistic approaches like traditional Chinese medicine view the universe and each part of it as a hologram rather than the more linear perspective of western medicine. Here is a blog written by an acupuncturist named Jennifer Kapraun, which explains this view very well:

"Last week my favorite coffee shop was serving a blend called 'Hologram.' As I sipped from my cup, distinct flavors: blueberry, toast, sour, chocolate, bitter, would emerge and then recede and then merge again into the flavor we call "coffee." That cup of coffee was, in a word, heavenly. Drinking 'Hologram' made me think of one of the central principles of Chinese Medicine: each part is contained within the whole and the image of the whole is reflected within the confines of each part.

A whole contains parts, of course. But one part containing the whole can be a more difficult concept to grasp. It is not a supernatural concept though. Empirical evidence exists in Biology: humans have recently (cosmically speaking) discovered DNA, coiled instructions for the entire body contained within each cell. And recently (in the scheme of things) physicists may have proven the universe itself is holographic, that is to say, information about an entire region of space may be encoded at its borders.

This foundational holographic principle (also known as the macrocosm/microcosm principle) enables acupuncturists to discern a complex image of how your body's systems are functioning almost instantaneously. If your acupuncturist has taken your pulse, looked at your tongue, or pressed points on your ears or your abdomen, you have seen this principle in use. The tongue, radial pulses, abdomen, face, and foot, for example, all contain a "map" of the entire body. When we press three fingers on your wrist pulse, we feel a reflection of how blood is moving through the upper, middle, and lower "chambers" of your torso. When we peer at your tongue, we see the temperature, moistness or dryness, swelling or mucus in different organs of your body. When we press on areas of your ear, we may feel areas that are sore, numb, or painful in corresponding areas elsewhere in your body. These visual and tactile methods of collecting information let your practitioner see where subtle changes in one area may cause the entire ecosystem that is you to become more balanced and healthier, or less.

Acupuncturists and Chinese herbalists have neither the perspective nor the diagnostic tools to zero in on single cause the way a biomedical doctor does. Your regular doctor will ask questions to construct a linear narrative or story about your disease; she or he may collect tissue for measurement and analysis, or they may even collect images (X-rays, MRIs) but only images of discrete parts, not of you in your entirety. Doctors' tools and theories make them great at identifying and eliminating single causes where such exist, but Chinese medicine excels when complex factors interact to create disease. Sometimes conventional medicine fails to see that a symptom may serve a purpose. At times, a symptom may be what is holding the whole pattern, the whole fabric of you together.

Observing this microcosm/macrocosm principle may be valuable to you in your daily life. What problem are you dealing with at the moment? How are you defining the problem and how is it defining you? Is it best to zero in? Deal with things in a linear fashion? Or to soften your gaze and let the overall pattern emerge? Swift action or subtle recalibration? Yin or Yang? Good questions to ask of any of every hardship, discomfort, or health problem we may face. The interdependence of the part and the whole is central to the practice and power of Chinese Medicine, and central, I believe, to making sense of our ever more fragmented world.

Some big ideas to ponder over your morning coffee or tea.[26]

Canadian scientist and environmentalist David Suzuki co-wrote a book with Sarah Ellis called *Salmon Forest*, which was also made into a documentary that explores the connection between wild salmon and life in Alaska's Tongass National Forest, the largest national forest in the United States. Wild salmon and trees have a mutually beneficial relationship. Trees depend on salmon, and salmon depend on trees, say US researchers. Fish

---

[26] https://triangleacupunctureclinic.com/blog/hologram-where-microcosm-meets-macrocosm/

corpses fertilize riverside vegetation, and the woody debris improves salmon breeding success.

The 2019 documentary, *Fantastic Funghi,* featuring the inspired mycologist Paul Stamets and many other experts, is a descriptive time-lapse journey that took fifteen years to make about the magical, mysterious, and medicinal world of fungi and their power to heal, sustain, and contribute to the regeneration of life on Earth that began 3.5 billion years ago. It brilliantly reveals the fascinating world of mushrooms and our interdependence on them. [27] For example, when we think of mushrooms, we visualize the fruit of the mushroom above the ground level; however, the vast and complex root system of mushrooms called the mycelium can be compared to the neural network of our brain and nervous system in its structure and capacity to transmit information that literally allows trees to communicate with each other and their surrounding environment. Interestingly, the medicinal effects of various species of mushrooms "include hericenones, erinacines, scabronines, and dictyophorines—a series of compounds that could contribute to the growth of neurons (brain cells). Substances derived from edible mushrooms could also inhibit the production of beta-amyloid and phosphorylated tau, two toxic proteins whose over-accumulation in the brain coincides with the development of Alzheimer's and other forms of dementia.

---

[27] *Fantastic Fungi*, a film by Louie Schwartzberg, 2019, Netflix

In the future, the researchers would like to conduct a randomized controlled trial, testing the effect of ET and other plant-derived compounds on brain health—specifically verifying their protective role against cognitive decline."[28] Even "magic mushrooms," which we have avoided because they are toxic if consumed in large quantities or considered illicit drugs because they have been used recreationally in non-toxic doses for their mind-expanding effects, are now being researched for their capacity to "re-wire" our brain in micro dose protocols. Ironically, instead of making us incoherent, they can help us become more coherent in our mental, physical, and emotional functioning. "Re-wiring" the brain refers to the recent discovery that our brains have plasticity or the capacity to regenerate functions. Re-wiring not only allows us to recover lost or impaired functions, like vision and hearing but can allow us to think differently. How we think, perceive our world, and react or respond to who or what we interact with is conditioned by how our neurons have connected or "wired" together to process our experiences. Re-wiring allows us to think out of the box of our habitual mindsets.

So, when we use the term "plant medicine," we need to broaden our understanding not just to mean how we can use them to heal symptoms and cure physical diseases but how they can teach our body-minds to operate more functionally and harmoniously that not only benefits us as individuals but as an interactive society. For example, it has been found that mind-altering plants

---

[28] medicalnewstoday.com/articles/324710#A-dramatic-effect-on-cognitive-decline?

play an important role in effectively healing depression.

Depression is not just a psycho-physical condition. It is also how we experience and perceive our world, inner and outer. It can be fairly argued that our society is dealing with a collective depression that both limits our enjoyment of life and fosters a lot of destructive behavior.

Addiction is both self-destructive and contributes significantly to the destruction of the fabric of our society. It has been down for some time that plant medicine can cure addiction:

"Substances known as psychedelics, hallucinogens and entheogens have been employed in ethnomedical traditions for thousands of years, but after promising uses in the 1950's and 1960's they were largely prohibited in medical treatment and human research starting in the 1970's as part of the fallout from the war on drugs. Nonetheless, there are a number of studies which suggest that these substances have potential applications in the treatment of addictions. While these substances are generally classified as Schedule I, alleging no established medical uses and a high drug abuse potential, there is nonetheless evidence indicating they might be safe and effective tools for short term interventions in addictions treatment. Evidence suggests that the psychedelics have a much greater safety profile than the major addictive drugs, having extremely low levels of mortality, and producing little if any physical dependence. This paper reviews studies evaluating the use of LSD, peyote, ibogaine and ayahuasca in the treatment of dependencies and the possible mechanisms underlying the indications of effectiveness. Evidence suggests that these substances help assist recovery from drug dependency through a variety of therapeutic mechanisms, including a notable "after-glow" effect that in part reflects their action on the serotonin neurotransmitter system. Serotonin has been long recognized as central to psychedelics' well-known phenomenological, physical, emotional and cognitive dynamics. These serotonin-based dynamics are directly relevant to treatment of addiction because of depressed serotonin levels found in addict populations, as well as the role of serotonin as a neuromodulator affecting many other neurotransmitter systems.[29]

To put this in perspective, I am not suggesting that we rely on plant medicine to take care of all our problems. Nature works with our participation, so we have a responsible role in how we interact with it. In my case, before I discovered and took up the practice of meditation in my early twenties, I used psychedelics for a few years in my search for meaning and fulfillment in my life. I met a meditator while under the influence of mescaline, the synthetic form of peyote, and he was able to tune into the expanded state of consciousness that I was experiencing. He introduced me to the practice of meditation, and soon after, I gave up using substances to access heightened states of awareness. It was not until many years later that I occasionally shared a joint of cannabis with others, and I didn't have any attraction to trying more powerful mind-altering substances until

---

[29] https://pubmed.ncbi.nlm.nih.gov/25563446/v

more recently. I should mention that I have been doing deep breathing exercises as well as my daily practice of meditation and basic pranayama breathwork for the past several years and that deep breathing creates hormonal changes, including the release of dimethyltryptamine or DMT, which is a hallucinogenic tryptamine chemical that belongs to a class of psychedelics that includes LSD, psilocybin, and ayahuasca. "It is abundant in nature and found in numerous plants and animals, and even in our own bodies. DMT is the only psychedelic substance known to occur naturally in the human body, and studies have detected DMT in human blood, brain, and cerebrospinal fluid."[30] As breathwork experiences and benefits often parallel those of DMT and other psychedelic plant medicines, I felt no need to ingest or smoke an external substance for my personal healing and evolution. However, in recent years, I have been called to experiment with DMT both from animal and plant sources and have found that they have made me aware of how interdependent I and all creatures are with nature.

I have included plant medicine in sharing my thoughts about environmental consciousness because I believe our use and misuse of them parallels our abuse of our environment and each other. One man's food is another man's poison. This does not just refer to our different physiological constitutions. Nature can be toxic or nourishing, depending on how we interact with it, and the state of our physical, social, and political environment

---

[30] https://alchemyofbreath.com/does-breathwork-release-the-psychedelic-spirit-molecule-dmt-in-the-body/

today reflects how much we need to reconnect sensitively and intelligently with our inner and outer world. Interestingly, along with the disillusionment and discouragement that many of us are experiencing these days, what used to be demonized as toxic substances is now emerging from our collective shadow and being called plant medicine. Perhaps Adam and Eve have learned from their experience of eating the forbidden fruit of the Tree of Knowledge of good and evil, and with proper guidance by qualified and responsible stewards of our garden, we can heal our diseased souls and co-create a better world.

Education and Right Livelihood

Education and right livelihood are power tools in the toolbox of the artist of life. It would be misleading to say that right livelihood means earning a good living. For most of us, this means earning enough money to feed and house ourselves and our families. Within that spectrum, there are many levels of success, from those who are surviving day to day with minimal levels of comfort to those who have way more than they can use. In either case, we cannot assume that life is good. We also cannot assume that success, whether it refers to achieving fame or fortune, provides us with a good life.

No doubt, being so poor that one is not getting enough to eat, or proper shelter will make it very difficult to enjoy a good life. However, when we talk about success, we need to evaluate what we are being successful at. Success refers to how one step leads to another. Though it usually suggests a positive outcome, it would be more accurate to say that it achieves a desired result, which is not necessarily the same. We have heard that we should watch what we pray for. A good life is not just earned; it is co-created or cultivated. We need to plant the right seeds in the appropriate conditions and do our part to care for their healthy growth to reap the harvest. It is the same for a farmer, a businessman, a professional lawyer, a doctor, a teacher, a politician, or an artist.

Education is an important prerequisite for right livelihood. That may seem quite obvious if, by right livelihood, we mean a lucrative career, and indeed, our educational institutions have evolved to support that goal. However, universities were not originally intended to be career schools. Before universities, most advanced civilizations needed higher education to train their ruling, priestly, military, and service elites.

The first universities were in medieval Europe. They were schools of higher learning, combining teaching and scholarship and characterized by corporate autonomy and academic freedom. As they became more secular, they moved more toward training people for particular professions and crafts. The industrial revolution contributed to this tendency.

Additionally, universities offer an environment for creating, testing, evaluating, and applying theories to business, industry, and civic and community engagement. However, they are still communities dedicated to their members' learning and personal development. When I attended my daughter's graduation at my alma mater university, the dean gave a speech in which she referred to thinking critically as one of the primary goals of education. This inspired me and reminded me of a conversation I had many years ago with Joseph Heller, who taught and mentored me in the form of bodywork called Hellerwork, combining myofascial release, neuro-muscular re-education, and dialogue.

I had been considering another similar training that required six months of auditing, basically watching others being trained before participating in hands-on practice. Given my experience in high school and university, where I spent a lot of time dosing off in class, I knew that wouldn't work for me. Joseph told me that he did not use that approach. Ida Rolf, who developed the bodywork aspect of his method, claimed that one cannot teach someone a concept for which they don't have an experience. He also told me that the word education comes from the Latin *ex-ducere*, which means to lead out of.

Education is meant to draw knowledge from a person rather than put concepts into their head. I enrolled in his training, which provided me with a fulfilling career and transformed me personally. During the Hellerwork training, I was introduced to Voice Dialogue, which led to my training in this psycho-spiritual process and other related training. I learned far more about psychology in these courses than from majoring in psychology in my undergraduate university courses.

When I say that education is an important prerequisite for right livelihood, I need to qualify what

I consider right livelihood. The term is used in Buddhist teachings to refer to the fifth fold of the Eightfold Path to enlightenment or self-realization. The Buddhist monk Thich Nhat Hang describes it this way: "To practice Right Livelihood (*samyag ajiva*), you have to find a way to earn your living without transgressing your ideals of love and compassion. The way you support yourself can be an expression of your deepest self, or it can be a source of suffering for you and others."[31] It is interesting that Right Livelihood situates itself in the middle fold between the preceding folds of Right View, Right Intention, Right Speech, and Right Action, which emphasize ethical conduct, and the following folds of Right Effort, Right Mindfulness, and Right Concentration, which focus on inner connection. Thich Nhat Hanh wisely expresses this connection by stating that we need to be connected to our deepest selves in order not to cause suffering. It is not enough to follow moral codes or social ethics that we have been taught. We need to know ourselves and be true to who we are to live a life that does not compromise our essence.

Preparation for right livelihood begins before we are born. Whether we call it genetics or karma, we inherit generational trauma and its imprint on our perceptions and belief systems—what Christians call the sins of our fathers. So, when Thich Nhat Hanh says that the way we support ourselves needs to be an expression of our deepest self in order not to be a source of suffering for ourselves or others, we need to dig deeper. We cannot

---

[31] The Heart of the Buddha's Teaching by Thich Nhat Hans [Parallax Press, 1998], p. 104

change our past, nor can we recall what precedes our conscious memory in this lifetime, but we can heal the presence of the past through proper education.

The sooner we are introduced to critical and creative thinking that is not just a transmission of values, belief systems, and prejudices passed on through multiple generations but rather a perspective and discipline that allows us to cultivate an open and inquisitive mind, the more likely we can tune into common sense in the deepest sense of the word. From this connected intelligence that understands our interdependence with nature, indeed with everything that is happening inside, outside, and all around us, we are empowered with the capacity to conduct our lives not just from a borrowed rulebook or the trance of our entrenched belief systems and society's values but with the wisdom and compassion of the vision of Oneness.

Let me flesh out these rather abstract concepts with an example of how karma, generational trauma, and education can affect our choice of right livelihood.

My mother was born into comfortable circumstances in Paris, France. World War II broke out when she was ten, which shook her world. Her mother had Jewish roots, so the Nazi occupation of Paris was oppressive and threatened their lifestyle. They were forced to flee with whatever belongings they could gather and travel to a more remote location in the south of France. My mother and her younger sister were quite indulged with the comforts of life until then, but now they could no longer take that for granted, and they learned to fend for themselves without the presence of their father, who had stayed behind in Paris to fulfill his duties in the French government and other aspects of French culture.

Years later, at the tender age of eighteen, my mother eloped with my father, who was only a year older, to sail to New York and ended up in Montreal, Canada. My twin brother and I were conceived and born there when my mother was only nineteen. Our parents did not have the support of their parents, and my father was an artist painter who was more focused on his own interests than supporting his family and bringing up his children. My mother had to go to work and took a job as a salesgirl in a Montreal department store. At that time, the status of women was even less privileged in comparison to men in our society in terms of equity of pay and potential for advancement than it is today, so my mother had to work hard to make her way up the corporate ladder to an executive position, which was a rare accomplishment for a woman in those days.

On top of that, she and my father separated when I was five, so she had to assume the role of the mother and father in his absence. To her credit, she managed, and this allowed us to live comfortably, but her experience shaped her concept of what it meant to be successful. Put simply, for her to be successful meant to make a lot of money, and to manage that as a woman in a man's world required one to excel. So, when I came home from school with my report card feeling quite good about placing in the top five of my class, I did not get the congratulations I expected from my mother. I was simply told that I could do better. The message I got from my mother was that to be loved, I need to be successful, and success for her meant making a lot of money. I consequently became less motivated to achieve quantifiable results in my studies and developed a negative attitude toward acquiring money.

Of course, more factors shaped my liberal choices of studies, practices, and careers than my rejection of the business of making money as the ultimate goal, and I also learned that money per se is not evil any more than any other form of energy. I also realized how my prejudices toward money held me back from manifesting what I wanted in other areas of my life. The point that I want to make with this example of my process is that right livelihood is not just a means of making money, and to discover and determine what right livelihood is for each one of us, we need to educate ourselves, which requires us to not only learn about what possibilities are "out there" but what choices accord with our own values.

What are My Values?

How are we to distinguish our own values from the desires or habits that have been passed down by our parents, their parents, our society, cultural traditions, and what we have learned from our mentors and teachers? We cannot claim exclusive ownership of what we value. Our values are borrowed from infinite sources. However, as pointed out in the section on Voice Dialogue, it is fundamental to know who or which part of us is acting or reacting in response to any given situation. It is the same when it comes to determining what we value.

If we make a daily habit of checking in using the methods described in the section on Inner Work, we can first cultivate an aware ego that has the capacity to recognize the various agendas of the different voices within us. Then we are in a better position to discover what is our deepest value. I asked myself that question and got a clear answer very early in the process of writing Morning Pages. It may be revealed to you in a dream, in a meditation—guided or not—or spontaneously in that precious moment when your mind is free from the reins of its conditioned tendencies. This value is the foundation for manifesting what fulfills our deepest needs.

There are many programs and courses out there that can effectively help us manifest our goals, whether it be a career, a relationship, or a project, but the ultimate litmus test is whether our goal or project is in agreement with our deepest value, which is shared by all parts of us, all our selves or personas. A term that has become popular in several self-development and manifestation modalities today is the "authentic self." In my view, what is authentic or true cannot be partial, so it cannot refer to one self or persona in our ego complex with its particular tendencies or agendas. Rather it is the expression of our alignment with the fundamental value common to all parts of us that will not compromise our trajectory toward truth. It is also a work in process. Discovering our authentic self, listening to its guidance, and actualizing its directives is what I call walking the talk.

Personal and Social Responsibility

To cultivate a lifestyle that works for us, we need to choose from a position of awareness that is concerned not only with how we can manifest our needs or desires but also how we shall be affected by our choices and how our choices will affect others. Responsibility is not a fixed role or state. It is an ongoing commitment to align our thoughts, speech, and actions with our fundamental values. That requires us to balance a fluid and flexible attitude that can surrender to the winds and waves of change that life presents us with a steadfast commitment to honoring our intentions—keeping our ship on course, so to speak. The poet Kahlil Gibran beautifully articulates this balance in his seminal work *The Prophet,* describing the relationship between reason and passion:

> Your reason and your passion are the rudder and the sails of your seafaring soul.
> If either your sails or your rudder be broken, you can but toss and drift, or else be held at a standstill in mid-seas.
> For reason, ruling alone is a force confining; and passion, unattended, is a flame that burns to its own destruction.
> Therefore, let your soul exalt your reason to the height of passion, that it may sing;
> And let it direct your passion with reason, that your passion may live through its own daily resurrection, and like the phoenix rise above its own ashes.

I would have you consider your judgment and your appetite even as you would two loved guests in your house.

Surely you would not honor one guest above the other; for he who is more mindful of one loses the love and the faith of both.

Among the hills, when you sit in the cool shade of the white poplars, sharing the peace and serenity of distant fields, and meadows—then let your heart say in silence, 'God rests in reason.'

And when the storm comes, and the mighty wind shakes the forest, and thunder and lightning proclaim the majesty of the sky, —then let your heart say in awe, 'God moves in passion.'"

My teacher and mentor, Joseph Heller, used the surfing metaphor to describe the similar dynamic between surrender and control. A surfer needs to surrender to the wave but control his or her board. Though I only experienced the physical reality of that after taking up surfing in recent years, I have experienced the truth of the aptness of this metaphor in many areas of my life over the years, whether on the dance floor—with or without a partner—or in the dance of moment-to-moment choices I make in my life.

To translate this poetic philosophy into a more practical application, let us use the example of forming an intention to take up a particular practice. For example, after reading this book, you may be inspired to commit yourself to begin your day with a morning ritual of writing Morning Pages, breathwork, and meditation. So, you set your alarm to wake up at 5:30 am so that you can start your Morning Pages by 6 am, do your breathwork at 6:30 am, and meditate at 7 am. By 7:30 am or 8 am, you're ready to go surfing, run on a mountain path, or go to the gym or a yoga class.

As you turn off your alarm on your phone, you notice a few notifications that you check out, and 45 minutes later, you realize that you have gone down the online and social media rabbit hole. Now your mind is busy with thoughts about what you read or things you must do today, so you skip writing Morning Pages. You then realize that you have committed to a yoga class at 9 am, so you decide to cut down your time for breathwork and meditation.

Now, this can happen to any of us, and it has happened to me, so I speak from personal experience! However, let us look at the various ways we can respond to this situation.

For many people, this experience, or a few of them, will discourage them from keeping up their commitment. For others, they will rationalize that this is the level of commitment they are comfortable with and that one day, they might attend a full-on retreat to make up for it. For others, the experience might impress upon them the need to be uncompromising in their commitment, and they will make a rule for themselves not to get distracted by looking at their phone or get involved in any other activity before their planned schedule. Now, this last alternative is ideal, but what if, occasionally, one has an important appointment, or a friend wants to be introduced to the practice or a part of it and join you on a particular morning? Would you be willing to alter your plan?

Perhaps you may also be invited to participate in a practice different from yours. Would you allow yourself to alter your routine? At one extreme, these scenarios exemplify how one can rationalize a compromised intention in the name of surrendering to the winds of change. At the other extreme, if one is unwilling ever to break the rules that either one has set for oneself or that one has learned from a particular tradition, one might be erring in the direction of lacking flexibility in one's tight grip on one's routine. In either case, one is compromising the spirit of one's practice. We need to balance surrender with control by gracefully responding to the winds of change while exercising the discernment that comes with discipline, not to compromise the quality of life one wants to cultivate. The art of living is not about achieving perfection as a thing but practicing perfectly. Our path will include obstacles and detours. That is all part of the dance. It is up to us to respond with an aware ego to the twists and turns so that we can continue to flow with the river of life and be true to our purpose. One compromises that truth when one allows oneself to deviate from the path that one knows to be true for oneself. Ultimately, our own conscience is the rule-maker and arbitrator.

One of the ways that we can discern whether our choices are in accord with what we value most is whether they can pass the test of being both good for oneself and others. If my choice is bound to meet the standard that I believe others expect of me or a standard that I have previously set for myself but is not in accordance with my needs now, then I may need to question it. Similarly, if my choices meet my perceived personal needs but are harmful to others or my environment, I may need to let go of my plan or curb my impulses. Experience has taught me that while a part of me will protest or lament a lost opportunity, I have found that trusting my obedience to my highest value will yield, sooner or later, the most fulfilling result for all concerned. These principles seem quite simple on the surface, but our egos are complex and tricky. There is more than one self tugging at the strings that control our movements. Therefore, the practices that cultivate an aware ego, which, as described earlier, is not a fixed self but rather a living process, are fundamental. It is from that awareness that we can think, speak, and act responsibly.

Conclusion

As much as I have looked forward to this moment, I notice a resistance in me to ending this book. In fact, I experienced a similar feeling each time I ended a chapter. I suppose it is the dilemma of the artist. When do I decide that this is the last brush stroke of my painting, the last carving of my sculpture, or the final mix of my song? Ironically, creation seems to halt the creativity that engendered it. It is only fitting that a book about the art of living should be hard to end. It is a reminder that the essence of a well-lived life is to keep going with the flow, fully engaging our whole being to enjoy all the opportunities life presents us to be co-creators in the art of life.

It is not typical of me to be as concise as I have been in sharing the teachings and practices described in this book. This is an overview of practices I have been cultivating over the past fifty years and is meant as an introduction and invitation for you to dive more deeply into each of the practices and overall lifestyle to appreciate their transformative benefits fully. If you are interested in learning more about how I walk my talk so that you too can walk your talk, I shall be happy to share that with you in more depth in workshops and personal consultations that I offer live and online. These offerings will be found on my website: https://www.darylvansier.com/, and some of the practices I have described are taught by other teachers worldwide.

Namaste and Pura Vida

Footnotes

[1] http://www.bbc.com/earth/story/20170215-the-strange-link-between-the-human-mind-and-quantum-physics

[2] *The Power of Now*, Eckhart Tolle. Namaste Publishing 1997 Vancouver, B.C., Canada and New World Library 2004, Novato, California, USA. This is one of the essential books I have included in my recommended reading list to accompany this book both for its accessible instruction and the inspiration you will receive to practice living in the moment.

[3] https://www.susangregg.com/toltec-tradition/

[4] *The Four Agreements: A Practical Guide to Personal Freedom*, by Don Miguel Angel Ruiz, 1997 Amber-Allen Publishing; San Rafael, California

[5] https://www.ncbi.nlm.nih.gov/pmc/articles/PMC3992527/

https://www.ncbi.nlm.nih.gov/pmc/articles/PMC3253025/

[6] https://www.nigms.nih.gov/education/fact-sheets/Pages/circadian-rhythms.aspx

[7] https://www.artofliving.org/ayurveda-dinacharya-use-circadian-rhythm-your-body-optimal-wellness

[8] http://ashleyjosephine.com/ayurveda-circadian-rhythm/

[9] https://healthblog.uofmhealth.org/wellness-prevention/intermittent-fasting-it-right-for-you#:~:text=Besides%20weight%20loss%2C%20are%20there,motor%20coordination%20and%20improved%20sleep.

[10] https://www.healthline.com/nutrition/10-health-benefits-of-intermittent-fasting#section10

[11] https://www.health.harvard.edu/blog/intermittent-fasting-surprising-update-2018062914156

[12] *Get Up: Why Your Chair Is Killing You and What You Can Do About It."* - James A. Levine StMartin's Publishing; July 2014

[13] Laursen PB, Jenkins DG (2002). "The Scientific Basis for High-Intensity Interval Training." *Sports Medicine* (Review). **32** (1): 53–73.

[14] Zhang, Haifeng; Tong, Tom K.; Qiu, Weifeng; Zhang, Xu; Zhou, Shi; Liu, Yang; He, Yuxiu (2017-01-01). "Comparable Effects of High-Intensity Interval Training and Prolonged Continuous Exercise Training

on Abdominal Visceral Fat Reduction in Obese Young Women". *Journal of Diabetes Research.* **2017**: 5071740.

[15] https://www.webmd.com/sleep-disorders/benefits-sleep-more

[16] https://www.webmd.com/sleep-disorders/benefits-sleep-more

[17] https://www.webmd.com/sleep-disorders/benefits-sleep-more

[18] https://www.webmd.com/sleep-disorders/benefits-sleep-more

[19] https://www.webmd.com/sleep-disorders/benefits-sleep-more

[20] Neckelmann, D. et al., Chronic Insomnia as a Risk Factor for Developing Anxiety and Depression, Sleep. 2007; 30 (7): 873-880.

[21] https://www.sciencedirect.com/science/article/abs/pii/S2352721815000157

[22] https://www.sleepscore.com/all-about-sleep-why-is-it-important/

[23] https://www.wimhofmethod.com/breathing-exercises

[24] *The Artist's Way: A Spiritual Path to Higher Creativity* by Julia Cameron; Profile 2020

[25] *The Dark Side of Light Chasers* by Debbie Ford; Riverhead Books 2010

[26] https://pubmed.ncbi.nlm.nih.gov/16979104/

[27] https://triangleacupunctureclinic.com/blog/hologram-where-microcosm-meets-macrocosm/

[28] *Salmon Forest*: David Suzuki, Sarah Ellis, Greystone Books Ltd, 2003 Vancouver, B.C.

[29] *Fantastic Fungi*, a film by Louie Schwartzberg, 2019, Netflix

[30] medicalnewstoday.com/articles/324710#A-dramatic-effect-on-cognitive-decline?

[31] *The Brain That Changes Itself* by Norman Doidge M.D. 2007, James H. Silberman Books.

[32] https://www.webmd.com/depression/news/20220218/magic-mushrooms-depression-relief-study

[33] https://pubmed.ncbi.nlm.nih.gov/25563446/v

[34] https://alchemyofbreath.com/does-breathwork-release-the-psychedelic-spirit-molecule-dmt-in-the-body/

[35] *The Heart of the Buddha's Teaching* by Thich Nhat Hans [Parallax Press, 1998], p. 104

Bibliography

Fantastic Fungi, a film by Louie Schwartzberg, 2019, Netflix

Salmon Forest: David Suzuki, Sarah Ellis, Greystone Books Ltd, 2003 Vancouver, B.C.

The Artist's Way: A Spiritual Path to Higher Creativity by Julia Cameron; Profile 2020

The Brain That Changes Itself *by* Norman Doidge M.D. 2007, James H. Silberman Books.

The Dark Side of Light Chasers by Debbie Ford; Riverhead Books 2010

The Four Agreements: A Practical Guide to Personal Freedom, by Don Miguel Angel Ruiz, 1997 Amber-Allen Publishing; San Rafael, California

The Heart of the Buddha's Teaching by Thich Nhat Hans [Parallax Press, 1998], p. 104

The Power of Now, Eckhart Tolle. Namaste Publishing 1997 Vancouver, B.C., Canada and New World Library 2004, Novato, California, USA.

Recommended Reading List

Man's Search for Meaning - Viktor E. Frankl - 1946, 2006

The Power of Now - A Guide to Spiritual Enlightenment - Eckhart Tolle - 2004

The Four Agreements - A Practical Guide to Personal Freedom - Don Miguel Ruiz - 1997

The Primal Blueprint - Mark Sisson 2009

Embracing Ourselves - The Voice Dialogue Manual - Hal Stone, Sidra Stone - 1993

Inner Work: Using Dreams and Active Imagination for Personal Growth - Robert A. Johnson - 1989

Man and His Symbols - Carl Jung et al. - 1968

The Artist's Way - Julia Cameron - 1995

The Dark Side of Light Chasers - Debbie Ford - 1998

Light on Yoga - BKS Iyengar - 1966

Fantastic Fungi - Paul Stamets et al. - 2019 - Also watchable as documentary film by Louie Swartzberg on Netflix

Salmon Forest - David Suzuki - 2003

The Brain That Changes Itself - Norman Doidge - 2007

The Heart of Buddha's Teaching - Thich Nhat Hanh - 1998

The Prophet - Kahlil Gibran –1923

About the Author

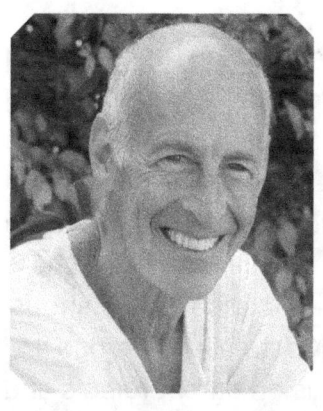

Born in Montreal, Canada in 1949, Daryl was introduced to yoga as a child and began to practice regularly as a teenager to successfully heal a painful congenital condition in his spine. Shortly after graduating from McGill University in Montreal, Canada, he was introduced to meditation and within months decided to dedicate himself to full-time practice as a Buddhist monk. He practiced Zen and Tibetan Buddhism for 11 years.

At 31 years of age, wishing to re-connect with the society he had left, Daryl left the monastic setting and trained in various massage and bodywork techniques to eventually become a body/mind therapist. He was particularly influenced by Hellerwork, a process of integration utilizing structural bodywork, movement education, and their relationship to one's emotions and attitudes. Drawing on his experience of the benefits of hatha yoga, Daryl gradually incorporated classical asanas into this therapeutic setting to help his clients contact and release tensions stored in their "body-mind", and designed specific routines appropriate to each person's needs to help them sustain the harmony, strength, and mobility achieved in the sessions. Impressed with the integrity of the Hellerwork process, Daryl designed a series of yoga posture flows corresponding to the various stages of the eleven-part Hellerwork series. This method came to be known as Divya Yoga and is recognized by the **Yoga Alliance.**

Daryl Vansier is an experienced meditation instructor and retreat guide, having meditated for over 50 years, training with Zen and Tibetan Buddhist Masters in the west as well as Raja Yoga Masters at the International Meditation Institute in India. In 1992 he founded Heaven and Earth Institute a healing arts center in Montreal Canada where he and other instructors offered classes, workshops, retreats and private sessions in Montreal and abroad. He closed his center in 2009 to focus on other projects and is currently based in Nosara, Costa Rica.

During his training in Hellerwork Daryl was introduced to the theory of sub-personalities and Voice Dialogue and this became an important influence in Daryl's personal and professional life. Daryl went on to train as a facilitator and teacher with the founders Hal and Sidra Stone and their staff. Drawing on his knowledge of this approach and related techniques such as dreamwork and Active Imagination and his extensive experience in the other healing arts he has practiced over a lifetime Daryl now shares his knowledge in workshops, retreats and personal lifestyle counseling sessions in Costa Rica and abroad.

www.ingramcontent.com/pod-product-compliance
Lightning Source LLC
LaVergne TN
LVHW021709060526
838200LV00050B/2582